D0834963

# THE PROFESSIONAL'S REFLEXOLOGY HANDBOOK

## By Shelley Marleen Hess

Blue Peel non Surgical Face L. Ft $60
ne VAATINE
1-800-451-1410S

## Online Services

**Delmar Online**

To access a wide variety of Delmar products and services on the World Wide Web,
point your browser to:

**http://www.delmar.com/delmar.html**
or email: info@delmar.com

**thomson.com**

To access International Thomson Publishing's
home site for information on more than 34 publishers
and 20,000 products, point your browser to:

**http://www.thomson.com**
or email: findit@kiosk.thomson.com

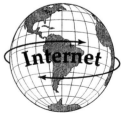

A service of  I(T)P®

# THE PROFESSIONAL'S REFLEXOLOGY HANDBOOK

## By Shelley Marleen Hess

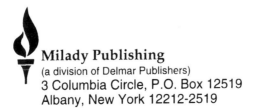

Milady Publishing
(a division of Delmar Publishers)
3 Columbia Circle, P.O. Box 12519
Albany, New York 12212-2519

## NOTICE TO THE READER

Publisher does not warrant or guarantee any of the products described herein or perform any independent analysis in connection with any of the product information contained herein. Publisher does not assume, and expressly disclaims, any obligation to obtain and include information other than that provided to it by the manufacturer.

The reader is expressly warned to consider and adopt all safety precautions that might be indicated by the activities herein and to avoid all potential hazards. By following the instructions contained herein, the reader willingly assumes all risks in connections with such instructions.

The publisher makes no representation or warranties of any kind, including but not limited to, the warranties of fitness for particular purpose or merchantability, nor are any such representations implied with respect to the material set forth herein, and the publisher takes no responsibility with respect to such material. The publisher shall not be liable for any special, consequential, or exemplary damages resulting, in whole or part, from the readers' use of, or reliance upon, this material.

**Milady Staff**
Publisher: Catherine Frangie
Acquisitions Editor: Joseph Miranda
Project Editor: Annette Downs Danaher
Production Manager: Brian Yacur
Production and Art/Design Coordinator: Suzanne Nelson

COPYRIGHT © 1997
Milady Publishing
(a division of Delmar Publishers)
an International Thomson Publishing company  I(T)P

Printed in the United States of America
Printed and distributed simultaneously in Canada

**For more information, contact:**
Milady Publishing
3 Columbia Circle , Box 12519
Albany, New York   12212-2519

All rights reserved. No part of this work covered by the copyright hereon may be reproduced or used in any form or by any means—graphic, electronic, or mechanical, including photocopying, recording, taping, or information storage and retrieval systems—without the written permission of the publisher.

   3   4   5   6   7   8   9   10    XXX    02   01

**Library of Congress Cataloging-in-Publication Data**

Hess, Shelley, 1954 –
     The professionals' reflexology handbook / by Shelley Marleen Hess.
        p.      cm.
     Includes index.
     ISBN: 1-56253-334-7
     1. Reflexotherapy —Handbooks, manuals, etc..   I. Title
RM723.R43H47   1996                                  95-48218
615.8'22 —dc20                                         CIP

# *Dedication*

I want to dedicate this book to some very special people. The first is my mother and "Guardian Angel." She has been a shining inspiration in my life.

Second is my closest friend, Ted Hampton. Thanks for listening to me during the entire process of writing this book. You never made me feel that I was burdening you.

A very special thank you goes to my sister, Jacqueline Hess, who kept me on track with my writing schedule and provided constant positive reinforcement at all hours, every day. I couldn't have done it without you!

# Contents

## PART I   The Professional Reflexologist

### Chapter One

### Chapter Two

## Chapter Six

# PART III   The Business of Reflexology

## Chapter Seven

# PART IV   Appendices

## *Appendix A*

## *Appendix B*

# Acknowledgments

During the past seventeen years I have had the opportunity to work with several different professional reflexologists. One of the best is Mr. Lynn Nelson, who has developed one of the most unique and best systems in current history. I want to acknowledge his contribution to the advancement of the profession.

I also want to thank Mr. Joseph Miranda from Milady Publishing Company for requesting that I write this book. He explained that it was needed to help others in the beauty industry. I also want to acknowledge the other staff members who were instrumental in putting this book together: Annette Downs Danaher and Marlene Pratt. Both women were invaluable to me during the writing of this book and the Salon Ovations *Guide to Aromatherapy*.

# *Foreword*

This book was written exclusively for you. It provides you with a step-by-step, practical way to bring a state of well-being to your clients. This will translate into better and more productive beauty care and very quickly will bring in more satisfied clients and more sales.

Reflexology is nearly 5,000 years old. First practiced in the Orient, and later in Egypt, it involves the massaging of specific areas of the hands and feet, which represent other parts of the body. Areas of the head, for example, are represented in the toes and the fingertips. There are corresponding areas on the soles of the feet and the palms of the hands for internal organs and other bodily systems. Proper massage and manipulation of these areas bring about feelings of relaxation and the relief of stress. Reflexology has become an essential tool in the advancement of the already exciting field of beauty care.

The amount of information we have available on reflexology has doubled and redoubled as we have become more aware of the natural healing powers of the body. The holistic approach to medicine has now expanded to the holistic approach to beauty care. It took an immensely talented writer, lecturer, and practitioner to pull together the material in this book. Shelley Hess, author of eight books, several translated into other languages, studied herbal medicine and reflexology with Madame Chei, a Chinese healer, for 4 years before she practiced these Chinese healing methods. After working and studying with experts in the field for more than 17 years, she has organized her knowledge of reflexology and offered it to us in this easy to read, easy to understand, and easy to apply workbook. What I like about Ms. Hess's book is the detail and insight she brings to the field. But, as a psychologist, I also appreciate her recognition of the limits of the work that can and should be done in a salon. She states, quite correctly, that some problems are outside the scope of beauty practitioners. Nonetheless, you can perform many procedures in the interest of your clients and these are clearly detailed. You need spend only a few minutes a day in conscientious study. The results will be apparent immediately.

—Dr. Neal Wiseman

Inside the womb, sound, light, smells, and tastes are suppressed. This suppression accelerates one sense, touch. The skin is the largest organ and must begin its growing process above all others. The shell we call skin holds us together. It is our primary sense and our first response to heat and cold, pain and pleasure, soft and rough, and sharp and blunt. It is an amazing organ.

This primal sense is a healing sense. Studies prove that premature infants who are touched grow 50% faster than those left untouched. Is it any wonder we hold our loved ones' hands in time of need?

Ignorance of reflexology has brought you to this book, which will either give you all the answers you have sought or inspire you to learn more.

As you read this primer of reflexology, use all of your senses to grasp the concepts. Use all of your senses to comprehend the application. Use all of your senses to help others.

—Lynn Nelson

# Notes from the Author

This book has been created to assist those in the beauty industry to better understand what reflexology is and give professionals a working guide to assist them in performing reflexology as an additional service to their clientele.

I have studied with a master of reflexology for 4 years. My personal trainer had used reflexology professionally for over 4 decades. For over 17 years, I have used my skills to help others. Even with all of this training, I am still continually improving and enriching my skills with other training. In my opinion, to truly master reflexology, you must take the studies seriously. In addition, professionals must dedicate themselves to practicing the art of reflexology daily for at least a year.

I realize that this advice falls into an area of controversy, with current classes and seminars that promise professionals that they will be able to perform reflexology on clients at the end of one day of training. This is simply not realistic. In the true sense of the word, it is blatant misrepresentation of what it takes to master the science of reflexology.

I recommend that you try to read this book, cover to cover. Then, you should set up a schedule of working parts of the reflexology program every single day for a month. To become good at reflexology takes practice, practice, and more practice.

Begin with one part of the reflective zones, the ears or hands or feet. Get really comfortable with exploring the meridians in that one body part. Study the chart of that region and choose 1 to 3 specific points that correspond to a particular body organ or skeletal system. Ask your friends if they will allow you to feel that chosen area. Once you know that you can zero in on anyone's meridian point, you are ready to begin training yourself for the next phase, the implementation phase, or the actual treatment session. When you are ready, begin to work on clients.

My trainer offered this advice: "If you want to dabble in reflexology, then work on your friends and family whenever you get a moment. If you really want to become a reflexologist, then start in one area of concentration, fine tune your senses to be able to detect the slightest differences in that area in all of your friends and family before you begin to work on clients for a living."

What my trainer did for me was to begin my training in the area of elimination—the points on the foot for the bladder, colon, intestinal tract, sinuses, ovaries, and prostate. The latter two dealt with the reproductive system and the fluid that is eliminated. My trainer had me evaluate daily five people whom she preselected. We recorded all the findings on each client profile she read and cross-checked my evaluations with her own. We did this daily routine for 6 months.

I recommend that you adopt part of this policy as you begin the journey to become the best reflexologist in your community. Good luck! I hope that I will have been a welcome part of your career.

# Introduction

The human body has a remarkable ability to heal itself. The process of **cellular rejuvenation** mystifies and excites researchers. Reflexologists know the body sends strong messages about how well the process of cellular renewal is doing. The human body also reveals areas of weakness that need additional support. It is by understanding the internal communication system that the reflexologist does the most incredible work.

As a professional reflexologist, you can get all the signals back in sequence, inform clients what areas need attention, and lastly but most importantly get them to return to have you work with them to restore or improve their health.

What this book will **not** do is offer the reader information relating to major medical problems. Other books on reflexology attempt to support the idea that reflexologists have the power to help the body heal itself from cancer, diabetes, high blood pressure, and other diseases and conditions. I do not accept or reject the idea that reflexology can provide such difficult solutions to these life-threatening situations. It is simply my opinion that the reflexologist within the beauty industry should never attempt to practice such treatments. To do so could result in legal difficulties for which the reflexologist could be severely penalized. A career could end in shambles. However, the areas covered in this book will not cause the reflexologist such difficulties.

The material set forth in this book was designed exclusively to meet the needs of the beauty professional. It has considered various elements found within the beauty industry and applied caution and detail for the respect of the professional, the industry, and the client alike.

I was trained by a Chinese woman who used reflexology in her medical practice for more than 40 years. As a student of this incredible holistic health practitioner, I learned a great deal about the medical uses of reflexology and have used the reflexology system in the beauty field for more than 17 years. Although many times I was tempted to use the medical training given to me, I never crossed into the medical arena inside of the salon. Never once has there been a cause for alarm. This book was created to have that historical track record repeat itself for you.

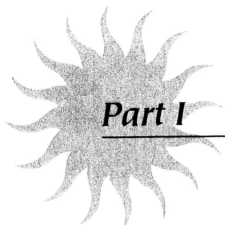

# Part I

# THE
# PROFESSIONAL
# REFLEXOLOGIST

# *Chapter One*

## WHAT IS REFLEXOLOGY?

## *Overview*

This chapter introduces the entire concept of reflexology and breaks down the various elements of the body as they relate to the process. It provides you with the information to begin understanding how to use reflexology in your professional career.

## *Introduction*

For centuries in the Orient, reflexology was the chosen source to evaluate the health of patients. Reflexology was the selected tool to create balance and harmony for the patient. In the last 25 years, reflexology has gained wide acceptance in our industry.

If used properly, reflexology can offer wonderful relief for the minor discomforts of daily life. Headaches, backaches, stomach distress, indigestion, constipation, and menstrual cramps are just some of the normal problems that can be relieved through the manipulations of reflexology.

Reflexology is not a substitute for normal medical care; it is rather a holistic health support system.

### An Explanation of Terms

The word "reflexology" has two parts—the root "reflex" and the suffix "ology." The suffix is easier to explain because "ology" at the end of a word means "the study of."

Thus, reflexology is the study of the reflexes. The root "reflex" does not refer to the muscle reflexes found in the area around the elbow and knee. During a routine doctor's examination a test of reflexes is to strike your elbow and kneecap with a rubber mallet to force your arm or lower leg to jerk involuntarily. The word "reflex" in this instance means reaction.

The use of the root "reflex" in the word reflexology refers to the reaction of the meridian points found throughout the body. **Meridian points** are highly sensitive nerve endings that send messages back to the brain. Through developed sensory pathways, they reveal what is going on inside the body. Another way to describe their ability to detect what is going on inside is to say that they act as a "reflex" to the internal system of the body. They are also called **reflex center points**.

Therefore, **reflexology** is the study of the reaction of the meridian points of the body. It is also the science of understanding the meridians themselves and the exact methods used to create balance within the internal system of the body by interceding and sending a new message back to the brain through the meridian points. Reflexology is also called zone therapy because it uses the various zones or meridian points on the body.

Although widely ignored by the medical profession, reflexology was respected by the holistic health practitioners and masseuses and masseurs for generations. As more medical doctors turn to alternative medicine, reflexology has become more interesting to them.

## The History of Reflexology

The science of reflexology is thousands of years old, dating back to at least 2500 BC. Early in its development, reflexology was used to handle all the health care issues of the people. Holistic healers chose the method to evaluate the patient, as it is now expected of physicians to take blood pressure readings or listen to the heart and lungs through a stethoscope during a routine office visit. In current terms, reflexology was the radiology, computed tomography, and magnetic resonance imaging of ancient times. It was the tool to determine what was happening inside the body.

In ancient times, an apprentice would travel with the master to learn the intricacies of the techniques. The apprentice was required to follow along as the expert skillfully went through the evaluation process. If the apprentice had at least a year's worth of outside observation, the expert would then have the student go through the same procedure. The expert would perform the treatment while the student recorded the suggested approach. The student's chosen treatment would be compared with the one performed by the expert. Once the student's recorded treatment matched the expert's selection, the student was allowed to perform minor treatments on the patients.

This is still the best kind of training for all the holistic approaches. However, it is no longer practical. Books such as this one allow readers to learn at their own pace. Repetition is part of the learning process. Any experienced reflexologist would say that you are constantly learning as you go along. Even after 17 years, I find that I am still learning new approaches and nuances that influence my decisions on treatment methods.

Although reflexology was never designed for the beauty industry, over time and as technologies have changed, the ancient ways have come into their own again. Within the beauty industry, there has been a renewed interest in all areas of holistic health. From **acupressure** to **Shiatsu**, beauty professionals are seeking ways to treat their clientele with proven, effective methods. Reflexology is just one of the best.

## Reflexology's Interaction With the Body

Reflexology works to discover how the soft tissue organs and the entire skeletal system are functioning. Through trained fingers, the reflexologist can detect early warning signs that the body is struggling and can then help restore the internal system to better balance.

Another way to explain the reflexology interaction with the body is by examining the ways the brain controls sending messages through the body. The brain has more than 2,000 major centers to get the news out. These centers are "supervisors" who watch over thousands of workers. The brain is the "head boss," and the supervisors report what is going on throughout the body, that is, what is working well and where problems are arising.

One of the crucial jobs of the human brain is to fix the parts of the body that need repair. The brain has a priority system for dealing with body repair. The number one rule is, "Above all else, do not let this body die today." The brain adjusts the scheduling of repairs based on how severe the damages are. An open wound takes priority over a bruise.

> **EXAMPLE:** If a person has a minor cut and bruise created while packing boxes on moving day, the brain sets into motion the process of decreasing the blood flow to the area that has been cut, so that the person does not bleed to death. The area of trauma to the capillaries and the blood spilled around them causing the bruise to form will be taken care of over the next 3 to 10 days. The brain causes the area to retract the blood around the capillaries and the tissue will return to normal when it is completed. The brain registers the urgency to stop the blood flow around the small cut as more important than the seepage of blood around the capillary walls in the bruised area. This is an example of the priority system the brain uses to deal with the body's many parts and functions.

**NOTE:** Only during minor cuts will the brain be able to stop the bleeding without medical support and attention.

My trainer used the analogy of a switchboard operator at a busy office. One hundred calls come in at the same time, and the operator determines which call gets answered first, second, third, and so forth. With reflexology, you can tell which calls have been attempted but have been on hold for too long. It aids the body in putting all of its working parts in good order.

## The Two Phases of Reflexology

Reflexology divides the body into 10 zones, all vertical, from the left and right sides. Using the spine as the center point, each side has five zones. The right side of the zone represents the right side of the body and vice versa. The first zone covers the area up and down the thumb and big toe. The reflexologist will work on all the zones during both parts of the treatment session.

Reflexology has two parts, the exploratory phase and the implementation phase. The more skilled you become in the first, the more successful will you be with the second. When you first start in reflexology, the exploratory phase will have great significance to the success of the implementation phase. Do not cut corners in taking exacting notes during the exploratory phase and refer to these notes when you begin the implementation phase.

### The Exploratory Phase

This first phase allows the reflexologist the opportunity to discover what is going on with the client. The meridian points of the ears, hands, and feet reveal much about the client. With very slight pressure on any of these meridian points, a slight degree of pain might be felt. On others, actual pain may be involved. Then, on other meridians there will be no tenderness at all.

During the exploratory phase, you go through the zones as you seek out the tiny crystallized deposits that surround the meridian point. The deposits feel like sand particles. Some will cluster together, giving the sensation of a group of wet sand granules rounded and bound up. The larger the cluster, the more tender the meridian point will be. Because it takes time for the cluster to develop, the nerve pathway has been affected for a longer period of time. It also represents the amount of time the body has been out of balance. If the client's condition has developed over time, several treatment sessions will be required to bring about an improvement.

**Crystals.** With the first phase you are searching for the "crystals." They are not magical rocks; they are deposits of calcium, uric acid, and other trace toxins in the blood. They accumulate when blood flow slows down. During the reduction of circulation, the calcium deposits create the surface crystals. When you break them apart, you increase the blood flow. The process increases the body's internal balancing program. Having the blood flow return to normal is a large part of obtaining the proper balance.

The reflexologist seeks out a certain kind of tenderness that actually feels good, even though it is overly sensitive, somewhat like an expression of a good "hurt." The reflexologist applies firm but gently increasing pressure but always is aware of the client's tolerance as meridian points are felt. Then the reflexologist backs off the point, making sure that there is no pain or throbbing sensation once pressure stops. The pain in the meridian reflex lets you know that there is pain in the associated body part.

The meridian point is always round but the area of tenderness may take on a slightly different shape. It will always include the round reflex point. The reflexologist has to locate the entire area that is tender to map out the area that doesn't hurt around the spot that does. Developing a proper evaluation sequence is important. Using the face of a clock as an example to do the mapping-out process, mark the area that is tender and move clockwise away from the spot.

Careful evaluation and specific note-taking during the exploratory phase will enable the reflexologist to provide an excellent implementation process. A big mistake a new reflexologist can make is to underestimate the importance of the first part of the session. Do not rush through it. Without a strong foundation, the rest of your work will have poor results. Clients may believe that the implementation phase is the reason they have come to you. But both parts of the process are important.

**Other Theories.** The medical community as a whole actually discounts the existence of crystals. They are not detected in any radiograph. Although physicians are trained to understand a great deal about anatomy, they are not trained to deal with the crystals.

Reflexologists strongly disagree with the medical community's concept. Reflexologists are more holistic in nature, and willingly accept the fact that we have not solved all the mysteries of the human body. We will also accept that we can work with information without having to fully explain its existence.

## The Implementation Phase

The implementation phase or treatment session is the second part of reflexology. During this phase, detail manipulations are performed to offer release of the client's problems. Once you have targeted the point, you being to seek out the crystals. Your level of commitment, your ability to evaluate many different people's meridian points, and your handling of the crystals will determine your success in becoming a good reflexologist.

Because the entire treatment is noninvasive, the client enjoys the added benefit of not having any side effects, which are frequent with many traditional medical treatments. Even without side effects, having the actual implementation phase performed can be uncomfortable and sometimes truly painful. The skilled reflexologist learns how to reduce the level of discomfort for each client. Everyone's pain threshhold or tolerance is different. The professional reflexologist quickly learns to assess the sensitivity of each client.

The student must become familiar with the various meridian points found on any ear, hand, or foot. These special points have a direct link with the organs and skeletal system inside the body. This is the hardest and most challenging aspect of understanding reflexology. The better you are at evaluating your client's ear, hand, and foot, the better you will be in executing the implementation phase.

When a reflexologist triggers one meridian point, others around it will sense the trigger and slowly activate also. Because an entire section can be activated by one triggering contact, reflexology can rebalance the entire body.

When you work on a client, you must learn which meridian points are closely interconnected. It is advisable to work connecting points all at the same time. Working all the meridians will gain a better result than working just one single meridain point. The following list presents some of the interconnecting meridian points.

- The digestive system includes the kidneys, liver, pancreas, stomach, intestines, bladder, and colon (ascending, descending, and transverse).
- The reproduction system includes the ovaries, uterus, and Fallopian tubes in women, so the reflexologist would do all the meridian points on the woman's foot or hand.
- The endocrine system includes the pituitary, thyroid, adrenal, and thymus glands.

- The eyes, ears, nose, and throat are all connected to sinus activity. Just working on the direct sinus meridian will not be effective.

# Typical Scenario of a Client's First Session

Normally, your clientele will fall into three distinctive categories:

1. They have already had a reflexology treatment before meeting you and were so happy with it that they are delighted to learn that the service is now available through your business.

2. They have heard of reflexology somewhere before but they are not quite sure what it does. They are curious about anything relating to holistic health.

3. They have never heard of reflexology and are only interested in it because you have aroused their interest based on your long-standing relationship with them. They will try anything you suggest at least once.

All three kinds of clients will enjoy the session and all will be candidates for a series of long-standing appointments for your treatments. The versatility of reflexology allows your many diverse clients to enjoy its rewards.

## Questions to Ask Your Client Before You Begin Treatment

Ask these questions in addition to those that the client will answer when filling out the Client History form (refer to page 132). Conversation before treatment will make the client more comfortable; the Client History form should be put in the client's permanent file.

1. What brought you here? Is there a specific problem that you are having right now?

2. If you are having a problem, have you seen or called your physician about it?

3. How long have you been experiencing this problem?

4. Does your family have a history of this condition?

5. Have you consumed any alcoholic beverages in the last 24 hours? (All alcohol affects the circulatory system and will cause the session to be less successful.)

6. How much salt is in your diet? (Salt increases the toxins in the blood, increases swelling in the joints, and makes some conditions, like arthritis, more intense.)

7. Do you smoke? (All cigarettes contain some degree of tar and nicotine and both of these increase the toxins in the body. The level of nicotine will cause the circulatory system to work overtime.)

8. How much water do you drink on a regular basis? (The more water the client can tolerate, the more the body will cleanse itself, and the reflexology session will offer greater results.)

9. How much caffeine do you consume? (This stimulant will cause headaches and body aches to seem more intense.)

10. Are you currently undergoing any major medical treatments? (If the answer is yes, get the doctor's approval before you begin the treatment. Lean toward caution!)

11. Do you get reflexology treatments on a regular basis or is this your first time?

12. Were you referred by someone? If so, who? (Send that person a thank you note!)

You have to decide if the client has come to you with a problem that should be handled by a medical practitioner or one that you can do something about. Reflexology will be able to ease most discomforts from conditions that are within your professional arena:

- Tension headaches
- Mild sinus congestion
- Menstrual cramps
- Constipation

These conditions are not life-threatening and the body handles them with or without your assistance.

The following are examples of discomforts that would not be within a reflexologist's professional scope:

- Headaches caused by eyesight troubles
- Mild concussions
- Sinus infections
- Cramping caused by miscarriage

Use common sense when determining your level of assistance.

## Beginning the Typical Session: Preparation

**NOTE:** As in most holistic treatments, energy flow is an important key to the success of the session. This means that you cannot begin the session if you have a headache or are grouchy for any reason. Your negative energy will pass through to the client. Your hands should be warm. If you are not able to use biofeedback techniques to make them warm, run them under very warm water before you begin the treatment.

Place the client in a comfortable reclining position. Most clients enjoy watching you work on their hands and feet.

Obviously, working on their ears does not allow them the luxury of watching. Bright lighting is not needed or warranted during the session, but soft music is a nice touch. The more relaxed your client is, the better the session will flow. Have clients loosen all binding articles of clothing, such as neckties and belts. Ask them to remove their shoes.

Begin each session with two hot towels. Wrap each foot in a separate towel. Leave the feet wrapped as you manipulate each foot with firm kneading motions. This should take 60 to 90 seconds for each foot. Remove the towels and spray the client's feet with witch hazel or any other skin astringent lotion. (Using a spray bottle makes the process quick and simple.) Pat the feet dry. Now you are ready to begin the exploratory phase of the reflexology session.

On the average, a singular session will take up to 20 minutes during and after the end of the implementation phase to bring about relief. The messages sent through the meridian points will take at least 5 minutes to register to the brain and back again.

## What Are the Expected Results From One Treatment?

Depending on each individual situation, the results of the initial reflexology session will differ. The reflexologist must first determine if the problem that the client presents is chronic (ongoing and long-lasting) or short term (e.g., a stuffy nose caused by a cold).

If the client has been dealing with the problem for a long time, you will not make a big change in a single session, no matter how experienced a reflexologist you may be. If the client has been experiencing a chronic problem, then the reflexologist can expect to be able to offer temporary relief of the situation.

**EXAMPLE:** The client comes into the salon with a headache. The reflexologist must first determine if the client experiences headaches most days or just occasionally. During the session, the reflexologist would encompass working all the meridian points in the feet and hands to relieve the pressure of the headache. The client will have to come in for a series of sessions. I set up clients on a three-times-a-week program for 6 weeks for chronic troubles.

For the client with a stuffy nose, I would work on their sinus, eyes, nose, and throat meridian points during the first session. Then I would offer the client an opportunity to return on an as-needed basis. If the client comes in at the first sign of a cold, the reflexology session can provide immediate relief and reduce (not eliminate) the backup of the sinuses for the remainder of the week. The client is made aware of the opportunity to return whenever he or she wants the session repeated. Reflexology is better for the internal system than all the over-the-counter (**OTC**) antihistamine medications and nasal sprays.

Reflexology will offer immediate assistance to all of the conditions or problems the client brings into a salon; however, it will not make an immediate permanent change in these conditions or problems with just one session. As long as you do not promise clients a single "miracle session," they will not be disappointed with the results. They know that the condition or problem did not appear overnight, and they will not expect you to make it magically disappear. How you explain your methods and techniques to your clients will aid them in working with you to create a program of sessions.

## *Summary*

By reading this chapter the novice may have the feeling that reflexology is too complicated to ever be understood. That is a natural response. During the first year of my training, I questioned whether I would ever "get the hang of it." I can assure you that with patience and commitment to your lessons, you will gain knowledge and confidence that will help you in all phases of your career. Reflexology is task driven, and the amount of time you put into learning the various parts will be appropriately balanced to your skill level.

It may be easier to break down the areas into related sections as you go through the entire surface of the hands, feet, and ears. Remember the top of the hand, foot, and ear all relate to the neck and head. The middle of the human body is reflected in the center sections of the hand, foot, and ear. Lastly, the meridians for the lower part of the body are found in the bottom sections of the hand, foot, and ear.

Don't give up—practice, practice, practice!

# Chapter Two

## WHO PERFORMS REFLEXOLOGY?

## Overview

Several different professions can work reflexology into their services—estheticians, hairdressers/stylists, manicurists/pedicurists, and masseuses/masseurs. Each group has specific guidelines to follow that affect how it uses reflexology while working on specific clientele. This chapter explains the guidelines as they pertain to all of these professionals.

## Introduction

Check with your local and state licensing boards to determine if you need a special license to practice reflexology in your state. Many states require a massage license, whereas many other states have no requirements because reflexology has not been singled out as a viable treatment. Now, with its increased popularity, the authoritative state boards are taking a closer look at the legalities of reflexology.

When there are no specific licensure requirements for the ability to perform reflexology, anyone can perform it. Does that mean that it is so simple a task that anyone can do it well? I do not think that is possible. Within the professional beauty industry are four distinctive groups of professionals who perform reflexology within their chosen specialties—massage therapists, manicurists, estheticians, and hairdressers/stylists.

## Professionals Practicing Reflexology

The training for each of these groups provides guidelines as to how reflexology fits into their specialty. Each is unique in its approach to the human body. Left to the original teachings within the industry specialty, the effective results of reflexology sessions would vary from very poor to average.

However, with the popularity of reflexology growing daily, the opportunity for all of these professionals to gain additional training opens up the chance to improve their techniques and provide excellent services to their clients. The key to their success lies in their determination to learn the most and practice even harder.

### Massage Therapists

When massage therapists (**masseuses** or **masseurs**) begin their training, they receive extensive information on the human body and its functions. They spend months learning the muscle and skeletal systems. They are taught the meridian points for the use of other massage forms such as Shiatsu and acupressure point massages. Because their training programs include so much more than the other areas within the professional beauty fields, massage therapists become more experienced reflexologists than the manicurist, esthetician, or hair stylist groups combined.

Massage therapists can be creative in their approach. A reflexology session can be performed on its own, or often they will combine reflexology with other massage techniques, such as Swedish body massage. For the masseuse/masseur, reflexology can be a means to add variety to massage routines. Masseuses and masseurs are the only ones in the beauty industry who have this much flexibility with reflexology. During the normal course of working, they have access to the ears, hands, and feet of every client. They must understand how to work all areas of the body to bring about relaxation, which is just one facet of creating balance in the body.

Holistic health is the current trend in massage therapy training. Masseuses and masseurs are leaning toward this quasimedical area. In chiropractor offices, masseuses and masseurs are hired and trained to perform physical therapy treatments. They use reflexology as an evaluation tool for their treatment routines.

In the Orient, reflexology is used as the evaluation process for several different types of treatment programs. Some of these have been adapted in the holistic practices of today. The masseuses and masseurs are the ideal candidates for these positions because their basic training is the perfect springboard for these more advanced methods.

In Europe, health spas use reflexology as part of the healing programs set up for their patrons. Over periods of 1 to 6 weeks, patrons are given daily treatment sessions, depending on the detailed evaluation of their health. The masseuses and masseurs can work on the patrons for hours at a time every day. They achieve incredible results due to the intensity of the sessions and the frequency of the treatments.

In the United States, day spas are opening everywhere. From large cities to rural areas, they are becoming extremely popular. Masseuses and masseurs are hired to perform many of the intensive therapies. Reflexology is popular as a way to eliminate the stress and strains of the client's internal organs. With a limited amount of time, reflexology will get better results than the standard massage therapies.

Reflexology is just one of the ways to distinguish a reputable masseuse from those who call themselves massage therapists but operate other kinds of services. The **nonlicensed massage therapists** will offer Swedish massage as a treatment routine. Their interests do not require reflexology or any other holistic routine to be part of their service menu. For years, reflexology was the clue a person could use when making a call to an establishment that advertised massage services. "Do you offer reflexology?" would be asked to see whether it were available. A yes answer meant that the place was not a front for another business.

### Manicurists

During their training, **manicurists** study the anatomy of the nails on the hands and feet. Previously, reflexology was not part of the curriculum. Now, due to its overwhelming popularity, reflexology has become a symbol to separate the average manicurist from the exceptional one. Reflexology fits well into their business because they are handling their client's hands and feet on a regular basis. Adding reflexology services along with standard manicures and pedicures makes sense from the practical and the financial sides.

When a newly licensed manicurist wants to build a clientele, offering reflexology as an added service can really pay off in the long run. It helps establish the new employee in a positive light among the other customers. Particularly in nail salons, the clients become friendly with the entire staff because of the closeness of the work stations and the frequency of their visits.

In a business with a nail department within a hair salon, new manicurists will build a better clientele retention base if they are perceived as professionals who offer extra services. A great way to be introduced to the stylist's clientele is to offer "arm-chair" service. Because reflexology does not require any lotions or equipment, the manicurist can easily work standing at the stylist's chair while the stylist continues working on the same client. Or while a client is processing, a manicurist can perform hand reflexology sessions.

The reception area is another perfect spot for manicurists to build their business rapport. No customer likes to be kept waiting, so new manicurists can perform hand reflexology sessions while customers wait for the stylists.

This service does not have to be free; the manicurist and hairdresser can work out an arrangement to benefit everyone.

During a standard manicure, the manicurist spends 3 to 5 minutes massaging a cream, lotion, or oil into the client's forearm, wrist, and hand. Instead, the manicurist can do an initial reflexology session in about 10 minutes and charge more money. The usual financial payment plan for reflexology sessions is a dollar per minute. By adding 5 additional minutes per head, the manicurist can add $10 to every manicure.

During the typical manicure massage, an inexpensive thick cream or lotion is used. Reflexology should be done with little slippage. Another service that ties together well with this treatment is a paraffin hand dipping. In this treatment, hands are dipped in melted paraffin wax and left to dry. After a few minutes, the soft, dry wax is peeled off the hands. Once it is removed the skin is warmed, smooth, and soft, which makes the process of the exploratory phase easy to perform. Using both of these services as an add-on to the standard manicure makes your services stand out among the others. The increase in revenue is substantial also.

This is particularly helpful now that a price war has developed among nail salons across the country. The current trend has created a nail salon in every strip center on most major boulevards and intersections. The competition to maintain a level of professional standards as these small establishments advertise a full manicure and pedicure for $12.00[1] leaves the experts fighting for the proper working

---

[1]This was taken from a sign at a nail salon in a Circle K strip center on Tustin Avenue and Katella Avenue in Orange, California. The shop sign read: Nails, Nails, Nails. When I looked inside I saw two rows of nail stations. Each row contained ten work stations. The room was narrow and long. The walls were white, with no decorations of any kind. The salon did not leave a positive impression for cleanliness or professionalism. This style of nail salon is common throughout Southern California; in addition, Broward County, Florida, Baltimore, Maryland, Washington, DC, and Arlington, Virginia, are full of these establishments.

atmosphere. These expert manicurists can use reflexology as a signal of their commitment to their craft, their interest in their clients' well-being, and the level of education they needed to perfect their skills.

A distinct advantage that manicurists have is that clients come in to see them on a regular basis. A client comes in for a manicure every week and a fill on acrylic nails every 2 weeks; a pedicure is usually scheduled bi-monthly or monthly.

The relationship between the manicurist and client develops quickly. The level of trust is easy to establish and therefore allows the reflexology sessions to be effective. This is especially true because many clients need more than one session. Making the client understand the importance of several treatment sessions is not the real difficulty. Getting the client's schedule to fit in additional sessions can be the problem. But manicurists and their clientele already are working with a closer schedule of appointments. Putting additional reflexology sessions into them is easy.

Some top manicurists hire newly licensed beginners to do the nail polishing, in which case they might have two clients at a time. But that is as far as it goes. In addition, the cost of all nail services never comes near the prices of perms, highlights, and root touch-ups. Therefore adding the dollar-per-minute fee for the reflexology can mean a totally different financial situation for the manicurist than it usually does for the stylist.

**Pedicure Services.** During a typical pedicure, the manicurist spends 10 minutes massaging the client's lower leg, ankle, and foot. The purpose is to relax the client's muscles. Now the manicurist can offer a more complete treatment for rebalancing the client's system along with relaxing the individual.

As with the manicure, the professional has the ability to gain more money for these services. The typical time spent on the foot is 20 to 30 minutes. At a dollar a minute, the manicurist adds $20 or $30 to the ticket price.

Most pedicures start with the client soaking the feet in warm water. This allows the reflexology session to be even more successful. The soaking provides increased stimulation to the meridian points and clean, soft skin to work on. Because reflexology should be done with little or no slippage, having the feet moistened from the foot bath is preferred.

Another service can be added to the reflexology session on the feet. A paraffin dipping will provide stimulation, softening of the skin around the ankles and feet, and additional revenue for the professional. The combined duo will make your clients boast about your services to everyone they come in contact with. The results are fantastic for client retention.

The manicurist has the choice of performing the reflexology session on the hands or feet and sometimes can work on both. This has several advantages. The manicurist can add variety to scheduled appointments. The treatment raises professionalism and adds revenue to the business. Clients now have another reason to tell their friends about their "nail tech." Because clients become friendly with their manicurist, they spread the word about the business to their circle of friends and relatives.

### Estheticians

The current trend is for **estheticians** to incorporate the reflexology treatment into their facial routines. The drive behind this decision comes from the interest in offering more creative services. Estheticians are gaining position within the medical community too. More dermatologists and plastic surgeons are adding estheticians as key employees of their staff, which has made them interested in taking additional classes in many subjects, including reflexology. The information provided through reflexology training gives estheticians material that allows them to provide better re-sults for their clients.

The skin conditions that prevail on a client's face are part of the reaction to what is going on with other body functions. A prime example is the connection of skin congestion and constipation of the intestinal tract. The body will eliminate toxins in any way that it can. One of the skin's many jobs is to provide an outlet for the body's toxins. If bacteria cannot get out in one direction, they will find a way out in another.

Depending on the balance of hormones in the body, the skin has a direct reaction to them. Both male and female hormones affect the complexion. Through reflexology, you can track the reproductive system, including its activity level. The more prepared the esthetician is to handle the results from the client's hormone releases, the better the client will like it. The happier the client, the more the business grows.

There is a unique position that reflexology can play in esthetic work that it does not play in the other fields within the beauty industry. The reflexology exploratory phase can be used by itself as a tool to create a more perfect facial. The information obtained through this part of a reflexology session gives the esthetician essential information to custom design the facial treatment.

The esthetician does not have to proceed with the implementation phase of the reflexology session, but can just record the information on the client record and then proceed with the skin cleansing routine. Here are just some examples of what the exploratory phase can do for the actual facial. The meridian points can tell the esthetician that...

...the client's bowels are backed up.

...the client's sinus cavities are filled.

...the client is ovulating.

...the client's stomach is tender.

...the client's adrenal gland is highly activated.

...the client's lymphatic glands are working hard.

...the client's thyroid gland is under stress.

All of this information allows the esthetician to realize that the client's endocrine system is overworked and has a direct effect on the blemishes and blotchy complexion the client is struggling with. The esthetician can help the client deal with the problems and provide answers to the client's questions.

Reflexology does not change the way a manicurist grooms the client's toes and nails nor does it change the way the masseuse or masseur manipulates the muscles during a Swedish massage. It does not affect the way the hairdresser cuts the client's hair. Only in esthetics can reflexology provide information that will aid the esthetician in performing a facial. The real dilemma lies in whether an esthetician should provide reflexology sessions on the client for the sole purpose of performing a reflexology treatment? No licensing statutes specifically cover estheticians to work on the hands and feet of the client. In fact, some may actually restrict such work.

The facial room is a private location inside of the salon, and the only two people who are aware of what goes on inside are the practitioner and the client. Quite frankly, these two have no reason to talk about it to any officials. This does pose a certain amount of concern regarding how to advertise the service, or whether to advertise it at all. As long as the esthetician uses the exploratory phase of reflexology as a method to gather information to provide a better facial, the practicioner would not be in any violation. The esthetician would not be able to charge for performing the exploratory. It would be part of the client evaluation process, which is the beginning stage of every facial treatment.

## Stylists

One dilemma that successful stylists have is that they have multiple clients being worked on simultaneously. One client will be in the shampoo area, one will be getting a permanent and another a tint touch-up, while another client will be under the dryer with some condition pack heating up, and yet another will be waiting in the reception area.

This stylist will have an assistant running around trying to keep all the timers going off in some kind of synchronized fashion. The stylist does not have the time to be performing a reflexology session! The irony is that the clients would greatly appreciate the attention along with the benefits that the session would provide.

I suggest that the stylist hire an additional assistant to do just reflexology. It would be the assistant's job to perform the reflexology sessions on the client's ears while she is in the shampoo area and work on the hands while she is processing a color, highlight, perm, or deep scalp/hair conditioning treatment. Having an extra pair of hands will allow the hairdresser to book even more people, without clients feeling as if they are being rushed in and out of the salon. The dollar-a-minute service charge for the reflexology session will more than pay for the hourly rate paid to most assistants.

It also makes your service profile among the rest of your staff appear to be more professional. This may seem to be a poor way to create a cohesive staff team, but it is not a secret that all salons have a competitiveness among the stylists. An important statistic to remember is that it takes four times for a customer to become a client who will stay with you. To gain the customer's loyalty, you have to go out of your way to provide more service for the money. Reflexology fits the bill perfectly.

Reflexology can aid stylists when they are starting over in a new salon or having to move or relocate to a new area, town, or state. Once again, stylists will have to prove them-selves to a new group of customers. Offering the reflexol-ogy session at the shampoo bowl, or while the clients are processing with chemical treatments, will make a positive, lasting impression. Once stylists get reestablished, they can hire assistants to perform the same services they originally had time to do.

Although stylists are licensed to work on the feet of any client, it is not realistic for them to consider doing so. Dur-ing the normal routine of the business day, the stylist will have easy access to the client's ears and hands. Because the hands are the second most effective meridian points on the body, the stylist will get good results during a treatment session. It also takes a shorter amount of time to work the hands so it is easier to fit it into the normal routine pattern of working on a client.

**Stylists and Manicurists Working Together.** Most clients love having more than one person working on them at the same time. Having reflexology being performed on the hand can have the manicurist working at the hairdresser's sta-tion. No supplies have to be carried to the work station, and the operator can stand while performing the service. One additional benefit is that it gets other clients "looking on" while it is being done. I have witnessed the positive effect this has on other customers.

The real dilemma comes in determining the pay scales between the two departments. The income capability of a stylist verses a manicurist is not even close to being realis-tically balanced. As previously mentioned, the stylist can have five clients all at the same time; the manicurist is lucky if one client is soaking in a pedicure bath while the final stages of polish are being applied to a manicure/acrylic fill appointment. One successful solution for the two depart-ments is to have the manicurist and stylist split the monies generated from reflexology sessions performed on the stylist's client by the manicurist. That way both feel they are benefiting from the arrangement, and the client feels pampered.

## *Summary*

In a perfect full-service salon/spa all the employees work together as a team. They share in the work assignments and offer the client the ability to have reflexology performed by many different people. However, in the real world, personalities, selfish drive, and other elements create scenarios that will not make the client's reflexology needs rise above their own. Therefore, the type of treatment will largely be determined by the professionals themselves. Massage therapists and hairdressers have the most freedom based on their licensing requirements. Levels of expertise and availability of time should not be pushed aside. The client suffers the most if these are ignored.

# Chapter Three

## THE SENSE OF TOUCH

## Overview

This chapter discusses the importance of understanding how to touch the client's body. There is not just one way to do it right. As a professional, you must create your own special methods that will provide the best service to a large number of people.

## Introduction

One part of reflexology is very important to understand, but it has nothing to do with the actual process of the technique. It is, however, an intrinsic part of the success or failure of the business side of being a professional. No matter whether you are a manicurist, esthetician, hair stylist, or masseuse/masseur, the value of this part of reflexology remains important.

This part is the sense of touch, commonly referred to as the "good touch" concept.

### What Is "Good Touch"?

Our society has become closed to the idea of open touching of one another. For many reasons this ideology has proven to be necessary and has a great deal of merit. But it removes from our daily routine the "good touch" one human being can provide to another. It has nothing to do with sexuality of any kind. It has everything to do with the need to express caring and thoughtfulness through the ability to hug, caress, or hold someone.

The need to be cared for and shown affection begins in infancy. Research studies have been done on infants who are raised with all of their biologic needs fulfilled. They are fed, bathed, clothed, and provided shelter. They are not given any form of personal interaction nor is affection shown to them in any way. The babies grow up with behavioral problems and are not well-adjusted children.[1]

In many households throughout the nation, individuals never receive a warm hug "hello." If you were to check with neighbors, family, and associates, you would be told how busy everyone is, and therefore no one has the time to seek out a daily embrace from a friend, significant other, or relative.

Adolescents do not think it's "cool" to come home and hug their parent(s). They are too busy; they go to their rooms for their own private space and private communication among their peers. In fact, children over the age of 9 years probably do not make time to hug their parent(s) goodnight.[2]

Clients may have other stresses in their lives that will attack if not rob them of their self-esteem. One valuable tool to regain balance in their minds is the use of touch. Hugs are one of the best uses of touch for this balancing. But a warm handshake, using both hands to sandwich the client's hand, is also a perfect substitute for an embrace. I call it my "**esthetic hug**." It is a great way to be personal but not extend oneself into the client's personal space without being invited.

---

[1] This information was given to me through a child development class, *Child Behavior From Infancy to the First Five Years*, during my studies for my undergraduate degree at the University of Baltimore, Baltimore, Maryland, June 1974.

[2] Dr. Phelps at UCLA has conducted studies on the brain development in children denied touch. His research was recorded through the American Medical Association technical support system. His work was reported on "PrimeTime Live" on July 19, 1995.

The handshake begins the process of "good touch." The client gets the feedback that you care. From that moment on, your relationship begins to build with the customer. Customers will become clients only after they have come back to see you more than twice. It is never too soon to create the bond that will make the relationship last. If clients can come to you to get their needed "good touch," then they will develop a need for you that will last a lifetime. The need to be cared for and shown affection begins in infancy. As we age, the need does not go away; it only increases. The ability to fulfill the need becomes more difficult.

Several years ago, an ad campaign was created through the United States Department of Health and Human Services. Bumper stickers and billboards were created with the phrase: "Have you hugged your child today?" It was so well received that mock stickers were created with phrases of all kinds, "Have you hugged your teddy bear today?" "Have you hugged your _____ today?"(every breed of dog was placed in this question).

A whole organization was started that promoted "group hugs." They felt that everyone should go around asking total strangers if they needed a hug. They made up T-shirts that had a symbol of two hands grasping each other on one side and two people hugging on the other, with the question "Do you need a hug?" They were open to the idea that anyone could approach them for a hug.

Some people felt that it was part of the "Love Child" movement of the 1960s. No matter where or why they were started, it made people aware of the need to have others show that they care. Seminars were created by the group, where the attendees could spend a whole weekend at a retreat. While they were away with the group, they received plenty of attention.

In the real world of their daily lives, it was not so easy to find a resource for such attention. Then there is their reflexologist....

## How Does the Professional Fill the Need?

As adults face various trying events in their lives, they will share details of these events with us, during the services that we provide. While they are with us, we have the opportunity to offer a contact through our hands that will make them feel comfortable, appreciated, and cared for. During any kind of massage or manicure, pedicure, facial, or hair care service, the client has the chance to get a special hug from us. Some of you will feel comfortable with providing each of your clients an actual full hug or embrace. Others will not. But the "esthetic hug" is perfect for everyone.

The "esthetic hug" allows us to provide a physical gesture that shows we are interested in the client. It does not cross over the line of being too personal, particularly with new customers. It gives us immediate feedback on how the clients feel about us. Is there hesitation in the way they allow your two hands to encase their one? Do they try to offer just their fingertips to your outstretched palm? Do they provide a "wet noodle" kind of handshake? All three are signs that clients are not ready for us to get too close to their bodies. We need to be sensitive to their reactions, which may not be directed to us personally. You must remember that customers might not have any opportunities in their daily activities that offer a warm handshake. Their lives might not have any outlet to express warm feelings. If we come along with a warm smile and double-handed handshake, we might surprise our clients. However, once the surprise wears off, they will love the contact.

An "esthetic hug" also provides the initial contact that will set the pace for the rest of the appointment session. All of our services are personal. Haircuts, facials, manicures, and pedicures are all done within the parameter of the two-foot margin called our **personal space**. Massages are even more personal because of the total nudity required. Reflexology services are personal from the direct contact and from all the personal information we obtain about our clients.

The information we get during a reflexology session is not just light gossip or friendly chatter. We really learn a great deal about our clients and their lives. The ability to get so close is just one more reason why the "good touching" is a vital element in creating the bond and trust between you and your client. Everything we do with our clients is personal. We must always remember the importance of keeping what they tell us totally confidential.

## The Appearance of the Professional's Hands

When you extend your hands to your clients, it is important to have your fingers and nails clean, healthy, and smooth. Remember that your hands are a direct reflection of you. Who would want to be touched by a lobster claw? Or worse yet, a dirty, smelly, lobster claw? If you smoke, remember that the tar and nicotine resins stay on your hands. Make sure that you keep a nail brush handy to scrub under your nails several times throughout the day.

The following is a true story and will show the value of these hygiene tips. I was hired to work in a well-known skin care center in Laguna Beach, California. I was introduced to the head esthetician. During the introduction, I shook her hand and noticed that her fingernails looked black underneath. Her palm felt slippery and she gave the classic "fingertips only" handshake.

This woman had worked at this salon for many years and had a solid clientele. I was shocked by my first impression. What surprised me the most was her dirty-looking nails. In fact, at the first moment, I really thought her nails and hands had to be dirty. However, it was an azulene oil that was used for every facial treatment as the massage vehicle. She was accustomed to it accumulating under her nails and was used to the appearance of the black lines under her nails. It never occurred to her that others might see her hands differently.

Once I became part of the team, I mentioned my initial reaction to her hands. She and other staff members were surprised. It never occurred to anyone that the azulene oil would be thought of as dirt under the nails. They had been using it for so long that they actually did not see the black-looking oil lines on their nails. They immediately decided to put nail brushes in each treatment room and to use them after every facial. Witch hazel was put into sprayer bottles for use after every treatment. This removed the slimy feeling from our palms without drying them out. This story illustrates that sometimes we are so close to the situation, we lose sight of what clients think about what they see. We never get a second chance to make that perfect first impression. The appearance of our hands speaks volumes about our own self-esteem and how valuable we can be to our new customer. Our hands tell our clients that we respect ourselves, that we are the ultimate professional and worthy of our customers and their hard-earned money.

For each professional, nail appearance may vary, however. Clients will not flock to a manicurist who has bitten off all of her nails. Nor will customers come to one who has chewed all the skin around the cuticles. If that is the condition of the professional's nails, why would I think that such a person could take proper care of mine? Nail biting is a habit reflexologists should avoid!

Generally, masseuses cannot have long nails. They can not do the massage work with anything but short nails. A reflexologist can also be a hairdresser, esthetician, or manicurist. Longer fingernails may be acceptable for them. The current trend in the manicuring world is to put a full set of acrylic nails on every manicurist, as a form of personal advertising. However, to do great reflexology treatments, we cannot have very long nails. The "good touch" cannot be properly accomplished with clawlike extensions. Reflexologists must be able to apply firm finger pressure with the "pad" of the fingers. If the reflexologist's nails flow past the tops of the fingers by more than 3/8 of an inch it will be difficult or impossible to get the right contact points with the client's body.

For the manicurist or other professional who really loves long nails, an adjustment can be made to the "no nails" policy. Some manicurists will keep the nails on their dominant hand's thumb and index finger short. They can then file the nails of their clients without the concern that the file will continually clip into their own nails. The reflexologist does need to use both hands. However, keeping with this idea, the reflexologist could keep the thumbnails and index fingernails very short, while the other nails can be considerably longer. It is still not a good idea to have the others too long. Anything past half an inch would probably appear too clawlike for the comfort of a reflexology client.

## *Summary*

Providing a form of reflexology to a client is a personal encounter. As a professional it is imperative that you fully understand how to approach a client's body with respect. On many occasions your services will be offered to a total stranger. This situation requires you to present the most dignified and professional approach the customer has ever received. From the moment you greet the customer to the time the person walks out the door, you must be aware of how you physically interact with the client.

# *Chapter Four*

## LIMITATIONS PLACED ON
## THE REFLEXOLOGIST

## *Overview*

Because we are not medical doctors or practitioners, we must be careful not to cross into areas that are out of our domain. Reflexology was used by Oriental holistic practitioners for centuries before it became fashionable enough to be included in the beauty industry. Each profession has legal restrictions that must be adhered to avoid getting into trouble. This chapter reviews the most common areas of concern.

## *Introduction*

All reflexologists must stay within the legal limits found in their area. When dealing within the beauty industry, additional laws must be considered. Make yourself aware of the ones that fit your specialty.

### What Are the Licensure Restrictions?

As individual as each state is, that is how different each state's licensing boards can be. There are no set guidelines that are followed in any of the professional categories within the beauty industry.

## Masseuses and Masseurs

Masseuses and masseurs have licenses that allow them to work all parts of the body. Therefore, they have total freedom to perform all aspects of reflexology and they can incorporate reflexology with all other massage treatments.

## Manicurists

Manicurists are licensed to work on the hands and feet. Working on the ears is probably not considered part of their "territory." My personal opinion is that they would not get into trouble if they decided to do minimal reflexology on a client's ears.

## Cosmetologists/Stylists

Cosmetologists/stylists are licensed to work on the hands and feet. Although actual treatment of the ears is not stipulated in their program, it is clearly understood that they are part of working on the head. Therefore, all cosmetologists can easily perform all aspects of reflexology on their clients, without any concern over licensure restrictions.

## Estheticians

Estheticians/facialists/cosmeticians do not have any licensing "territories" that allow them free rein to perform reflexology on their clients. In fact, several state cosmetology boards would find reflexology out of bounds for any estheticians/cosmeticians to consider.

However, I know that many of them perform such services in the privacy of a closed facial room. No one sees them perform reflexology. As long as at least one manicurist, masseuse/masseur, or hairdresser is at the location, reflexology can be freely advertised. In the salon where only facialists are employed (or booth rentals), there would be a risk in having an inspector from a state board of cosmetology find out during a routine inspection.

Unlike all of the other specialties in the beauty industry, reflexology does provide the esthetician with information that will aid in the facial process. It can have a direct benefit in producing better results during skin cleansing. For this reason alone, it puts estheticians in an awkward position, forcing them to hide from state boards that they are doing reflexology in the facial room.

Learning about the skin takes a great deal of study, as does learning how reflexology helps in skin care. I am bothered by the many one-day seminars that are presented to estheticians as a way to increase their income capacity by adding reflexology to their lists of services.

First, it takes a lot longer than one session to really know how to perform reflexology treatments. Second, it flies in the face of licensing restrictions. In reality, estheticians are usually very interested in holistic practices and reflexology is one of the best. So it is possible that this imbalance of licensure and reflexology for esthetics will remain unsolved.

## Reflexology and the Medical Profession: Knowing the Differences

Reflexology is able to address many areas that fall into the medical field. All of the major organs are reflected in the hands and feet. Attempting to work on the meridian points for the heart, lungs, kidneys, brain, gallbladder, and liver is foolish for any nonmedical professional. This will only open the door to trouble that can escalate into legal battles.

If your client perceives that your treatment is being done in lieu of medical attention, you can place your client's health in jeopardy. You have to be very careful that you do not present information to your client that can be interpreted as a diagnosis. Nonmedical professionals can analyze; medical practitioners diagnose.

When speaking to your clients about their reflexology treatment, use the term "session." It sounds less technical and therefore less likely to be confused with a doctor's visit. Remember that reflexology can begin to take effect in as little as 20 minutes. If you start to send messages to the brain to begin working major internal organs, like the heart and lungs, you can put your clients in an uncomfortable position. Their heartbeat can rise and their blood pressure increase. They may have difficulty pacing their breath. If you do not prepare your client for a sinus drain, their eyes, ears, and back of the throat will begin to fill with the mucus and phlegm that are released during the implementation phase of the reflexology session.

Clients may come to you asking your help in curing them of a major problem or disease. They may feel that the traditional methods of medicine have not provided the solutions to their condition and that alternative medicine is the proper course of action.

> **CAUTION:** Reflexology is considered by some to be part of alternative medicine methods. However true or misleading this idea is, please remember that at no time are you part of alternative medicine practice! You are part of the beauty industry. You are using reflexology to relieve stress and strains that are going on inside of your client's body. You must never present yourself as a holistic "healer"!

It is hard to look into the eyes of patients with cancer and not want to offer some ray of hope that you can help. All you can do is make them feel calmer and more in tune with themselves. You cannot rid them of the cancer cells. This caveat also applies to all other diseases that are difficult to live with and painful to experience. For these clients, offer a warm embrace and an ear to listen plus a reflexology session to make them calmer.

Do not go into elaborate evaluations of their internal organs; do not make it appear that you are "seeing into" the cancerous organ or tissue. If clients are undergoing chemotherapy, it is possible that every part of their feet and hands will be tender. The chemotherapy medicine flows throughout the entire circulatory system. Light pressure will be best when working on these clients.

Remember that the human body is a very complex entity, and you must respect its various elements. Using reflexology can be an incredible experience or it can seem like a bad nightmare. Go slowly and carefully. Do not proceed to work on clients until you are certain that your techniques are solid. Practice, practice, practice on all of your friends and relatives.

## Contraindications

There are four problems with presenting reflexology to the public as a method of bringing about relief for minor internal disturbances.

1. There can be misinterpretation of the power of the treatment. You can mistakenly give the impression that you will bring about a release of discomfort and you may not be able to do so.

2. You could unintentionally give the client the sense that going to the doctor is not necessary. Never, never imply this notion! You would be acting irresponsibly to do so. The wise approach is to include the medical review as the first thing the client should look into. Working along with the doctor's review is always more effective.

3. Because you are working within the beauty industry, you must not use reflexology for any major medical condition. **Cancer**, glaucoma, **diabetes**, and lupus are examples of conditions

that need medical attention. You simply cannot work the meridian points to rid the body of these and hundreds of other medical conditions. It is important that you stay within the boundaries of normal disturbances in the body. Once you realize your own limitations, you can work comfortably with the power of reflexology.

4. Although it is highly unlikely, you could place too much pressure on the soft tissue of the feet or hands and cause mild edema (swelling). Or, you could break a toe by applying too much force to the meridian. Be careful that this never happens!

As long as reflexology is not used as the only method to address minor aches and discomforts of daily body functions, there are no contraindications. The normal human body will automatically attempt to adjust any part of itself that is "out of sorts." Whether you use reflexology or not, the internal system of the body always tries to heal itself. Reflexology simply gives the body an added push in the right direction. Because you are working **relay points** (otherwise known as meridian points), you are not at any time directly pushing or prodding on the actual tissue of the organ that you are trying to relate to.

Although it is common for the medical field to frown on what a reflexologist does, to show respect for physicians' evaluation techniques is not only the best way to approach a client's problem, it will (over the long run) provide you with more respect from the medical community and from your clients. It also will limit any legal recourse someone might otherwise want to take against your work. It also keeps the medical review boards from interpreting that you are providing medical treatment without having a medical degree.

## *Summary*

Understanding the limits when providing health care within the beauty industry is essential so that we do not have legal hassles with our clientele. There has been a trend to "sue first" in several states, especially California, New York, and Florida, just to name a few. As a working reflexologist in all of them, I had to keep within the legal boundaries when offering health care assistance to my clients. Make sure your statements of how your reflexology will help do not sound like a physician giving advice.

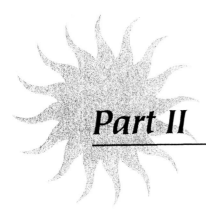

# Part II

# REFLEXOLOGY
# TREATMENTS

# *Chapter Five*

## TREATMENTS AND BODY PARTS

## *Overview*

Reflexology covers the full spectrum of the body. The science of reflexology gets into many different areas and conditions affecting the human body, inside and out. Each part of the body has a connection with the process through the meridians found in the hands, feet, and ears.

Learning the 3 treatment zones in reflexology is an effective way to increase your skill in the exploratory phase. Learn the treatment zones first, then explore how the message and receiving mechanism is set up with the rest of the body. Like the intricacies of a spider's web, reflexology has message relays that reach from the top of the head to the bottoms of the feet.

## *Introduction*

With reflexology, there are 3 areas that are filled with the zone points for evaluation and subsequent release for restoring balance to the body. The 3 areas are the ear, the hand, and the foot.

The foot is the area that has gained the most recognition. In order of ability to offer successful treatment, the foot is the best, followed by the hand and then the ear. All 3 are explored in this book. As a young apprentice in the study of reflexology, you are encouraged to work with all 3 areas during your studies.

# The Ear

We begin with the ear because it is the easiest. Its system of meridian points is not as complicated and it does not have a complex network. It is also limited in scope in its ability to assist the brain. For the beginner, it is easier to learn all the points and subsequent reactions they control.

Hairdressers, assistants, and estheticians can easily manipulate a client's ear during normal services. While the client has her head in the shampoo bowl, the assistant can work all of the zone points on both ears, before beginning the normal shampoo. All reflexology treatments are best performed with dry contact. No oils are required. The practitioner gets better control if the hands are not slipping off the zone points.

The ear does not have the same amount of reflective points as the hands and feet do. Unlike these two reflective zones, the ear does not cover a full range of internal organs. The ear does, however, reflect the body from the head to the buttocks, particularly the spine and the head/brain. Therefore, the ears are best used in reflexology for soothing stress and strain of the head and back.

## The Zone Points of the Ear

Because people have very different sized ears, the points will be easier to find on larger ears than on tiny ones. However, on the outer rim of the ear lie the zone points for the entire spinal column. The area where the top of the ear connects with the head represents the head. The bottom of the earlobe represents the buttocks.

If someone is having a tough time falling asleep, it is recommended that the person get into the fetal position. It is believed that the ear is the exact shape of the **fetal position**. Everyone can trace the outer edge of the ear to get the shape to sleep in. If the client is right-handed, have the individual trace the left ear, and obviously a left-handed

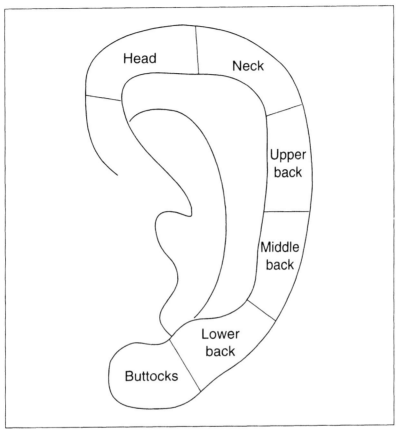

*FIGURE 5.1* *Zone points for the entire spinal column. (Points are the same for both ears.)*

person traces the right ear. If small children are having difficulty falling asleep, their mothers can assist them. All the mother has to do is help her child to curl into the correct position as the child lies down to sleep. I have known hundreds of people whom this technique has helped.

## How to Engage the Points for Treatment

The practitioner will use the dominant hand to perform the treatment. Only with considerable practice can you ex-

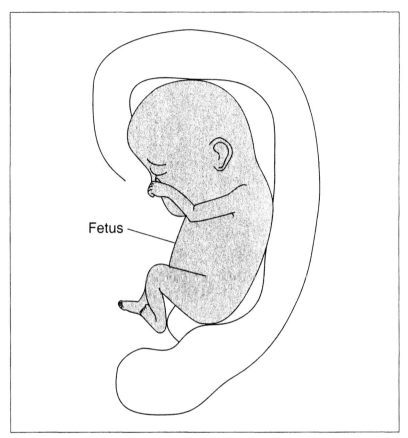

**FIGURE 5.2** *It is believed that the shape of the ear is the same as the fetal position.*

pect to be able to do both ears at the same time. Because the number of zone points is not as concentrated in the ear, it will not take much time to do each ear separately. Use the fleshy part of your thumb pad and support the back of the ear with your index finger. The client must remove all earrings before you begin.

Most people have very sensitive ears. A simple touch can cause someone to cringe, or it can create a tremor in a tickling reaction. Many people feel self-conscious about the

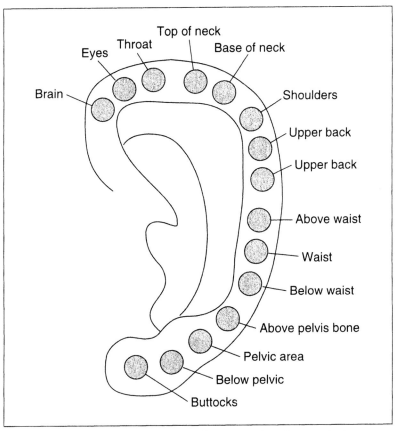

**FIGURE 5.3** *Refer to these points when engaging the ear during treatments.*

appearance of their ears; few people feel that their ears are attractive. For the most part, people take their ears for granted and do not pay much attention to their care or appearance. However, once you want to manipulate their ears, they become very aware of them.

Each treatment session always begins with the exploratory phase. This is important because you have to understand what condition the ear is in before you begin the implementation phase or treatment stage. Look for any area that may be cut or sore. Roll your fingers over the outer edge and feel for scaly skin; look for signs of eczema or psoriasis and check for warts. Remember you are not medically trained, so if anything looks suspicious, be cautious and do not continue with the treatment. Politely suggest that the individual have the ears checked by a physician. Reschedule the client for another appointment.

If the ears appear healthy on the outside, then continue with the exploratory phase of the session. Notice the way the outer edge curves and curls. Ideally, it is easier to perform reflexology on flat ears. You will not have the choice— ears come in all shapes and sizes.

Refer to the diagram of the ear. Using your thumb pad and the index finger, feel for the point on the top of the ear. This is the point for the head/brain. Work your fingers along the outer edge to feel for the rest. On the client's file, make note of any complaints of tenderness or soreness the client mentions as you manipulate the ears.

## The Hands

The hands are far more reflective than the ears. The meridian points of the hand are extensive and more easily accessible than those on the ears. Hands come in many different sizes; they vary as much as people's heights vary. Hands also come in different shapes, and their reflexes will vary.

The reflex meridian points on the palm of the hand respond to the front of the body, whereas the meridian points on the back of the hand respond to the back of the body. The spinal reflexes are smaller than those on the feet, but larger than those on the ears. The sinus reflexes are larger than those on the feet because fingers are larger than toes. The left and right hands have similar points, and each has points that the other does not. In addition, the hands are more exposed and need to be tougher on the surface so the meridian points are deeper under the skin. This makes it harder to reach the tender spots and more difficult to treat the crystals.

The reflexologist must determine which is the dominant side of the client. The reflexologist will begin to work with the **nondominant** side first. In reflexology both sides of the body are important. Both sides have energy fields. But in each of us, one side is stronger than the other. It is thought that we are left-handed or right-handed based on which side has the stronger energy field. When using reflexology to explore what is going on inside of the body, the stronger energy field puts up a stronger shield or fence that we must cross through. Therefore, we will get a better reading of what is going on inside when we enter through the weaker field. Thus, beginning the exploratory and implementation phases on the nondominant side will get us a better result. On left-handed clients use their right side, and on right-handed clients use their left side.

## The Zone Points of the Hands

Depending on state board restrictions, estheticians may or may not be allowed to work on the hands. Cosmetologists/stylists are allowed to do so. All manicurists and all massage therapists are licensed to work the zones on the hands. Next to the feet, the hands are the most reflective part of the body. Each hand has distinctive areas of concentration for treatment selections, along with similar points found on both hands. When determining how to begin your exploratory phase, the same rule applies for the hands as for the ears. Begin your investigation on the client's nondominant side. When you begin the actual treatment session or the implementation phase, the specific zone point may be located on the client's dominant side.

All the major organs are reflective on the hands. The entire skeletal system is also reflected. The body is represented from the top of the head to the toes in your hands. It

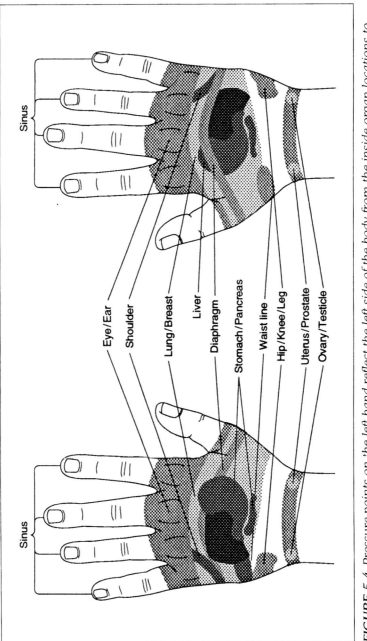

Sinus

Sinus

Eye/Ear

Shoulder

Lung/Breast

Liver

Diaphragm

Stomach/Pancreas

Waist line

Hip/Knee/Leg

Uterus/Prostate

Ovary/Testicle

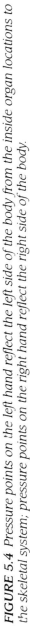

*FIGURE 5.4 Pressure points on the left hand reflect the left side of the body from the inside organ locations to the skeletal system; pressure points on the right hand reflect the right side of the body.*

begins at the top of the fingertips and ends at the base of the palms. The eyes, ears, sinuses, and neck are found on the fingertips, and the colon and ovaries are found at the base of the hand.

Many points on the hands are not within the range of our industry limits. Many parts of reflexology are closely related to the medical treatment of the body. If you are working in a nonmedical environment, it is my opinion that you should stay clear of any treatment regarding the major organs, such as the heart, liver, lungs, kidneys, spleen, and gallbladder. Full-service salons, day spas, massage clinics, manicuring salons, or skin care centers all fall into the category of non-medical facilities. While performing reflexology at these establishments, you should limit your treatment sessions to areas of relaxation and relief of minor symptoms.

We offer relief for minor discomforts. Some areas are easier to work with than others. The sinuses, ovaries, colon, and bladder are all areas that are often overworked but do not have actual serious medical difficulties or problems. We can aid the client's body and reduce the stress trapped in each of these organs. When the client comes in for regular services and complains of a tough period, or a sinus attack, or perhaps of constipation, you can offer assistance at that exact moment.

The hand charts are similar in the fact that they show you all the various reflective points of the body. One is the classic reflective chart. It is used by reflexologists who are in the holistic medical field. It is provided as a complete overview of the reflexology system.

It takes repetition and continual practice to zero in on a specific point and immediately be able to register what is going on inside your client's body. What will help you to master reflexology is to predetermine 1 to 3 different organs and coinciding meridian points found on the chart.

Then seek out all the people you can to evaluate their hand reflective points for those chosen organs. Once you

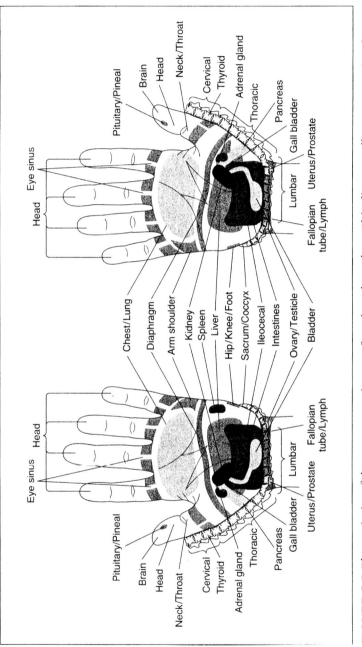

*FIGURE 5.5  The majority of the pressure points are found on the palms. This diagram allows you to visualize how the pressure points connect on both hands.*

get so comfortable with the selection and search mode, you will find your implementation phase is easy.

## How to Engage the Points for Treatment

You begin by taking the client's nondominant hand between both of yours. Envelop the client's hand with yours, while applying firm but caressing pressure over it. This sets the stage for confidence and control for the treatment. Repeat the process with the dominant hand. Notice that meridian points on each hand correlate to the same organ and skeletal part. Some internal organs are better zoned from one hand than the other. For other organs, it makes no difference at all. A few are reflective on both hands; however, they are divided from left or right based on their own location on the body. One example is the neck and liver. The neck is reflective at the base of both thumbs, whereas the liver is best reflective on the center palm of the right hand. There is a part of the liver reflective point on the left hand, but the right is a stronger point.

In working the eyes, ears, or sinuses, each is reflective on both sides of the body. Therefore, when manipulating the meridians on the palms and on the feet, remember that the left palm and foot handle the left eye, left ear, and sacs that lay on the left side of the face. The right palm and foot handle those areas that fall on the right side. The stomach is reflective on the left palm, but not on the right one. This is not the norm for most of the internal organs.

Getting acquainted with the chart is essential for your success in becoming a good reflexologist. The more you study and work with it, the quicker you will have it memorized. Do not hesitate to make copies of the hand chart for your clients. Giving them a chart of their own will add to their confidence in your work. It will make them feel more connected to the process and help them to understand how detailed the entire process can become. They will not be able to duplicate the work you do. It has taken you a long time to become proficient.

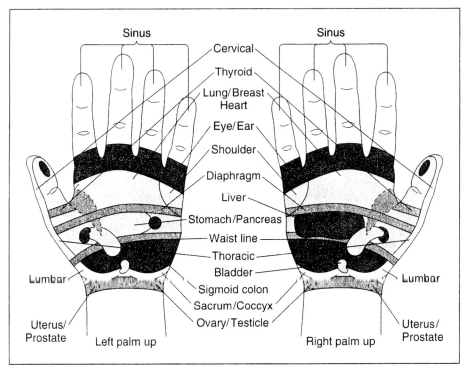

*FIGURE 5.6* Pressure points on the left and right hands, palms up.

Remember, the exploratory phase is even more difficult than the implementation phase. Be sure to take very good notes as you conduct the exploratory. You will be developing a relationship with this client, and it will be important to keep accurate records. No one is expected to remember every detail of each client without keeping updated files.

## The Feet

The feet are the most reflective of all and the most recognized worldwide in dealing with reflexology. The meridian points in the feet are the most sensitive because they are closer to the surface than those found on the hands. Zone points are stronger here than on the hands and ears.

They respond to treatment sessions more quickly than the other two areas. Part of the theory behind why the feet are so much more powerful in reflexology deals with how important they are to the balance of the body. Reflexology is designed to bring balance back to the body, and without the feet, the body would not have that balance.

## The Zone Points of the Feet

It is important to check your local state board restrictions to determine which licensed professionals are able to work on the feet. I am not aware of any state board that openly allows estheticians to work on the feet. However, I am personally aware that short seminars are being offered to them for the purpose of incorporating the service into their salon work. What goes on behind a closed door is none of my business. Perhaps that is also the opinion of the state boards. All massage therapists, manicurists, and most cosmetologists are allowed to work on the feet.

One of the charts shows all the meridian zone points for a complete reflexology treatment. It is important to remember that as beauty professionals, we should use the chart that highlights the areas that fall within our industry limits.

The body is reflective on the foot beginning from the top to the bottom. I recommend that we work on the areas of the body that deal with the elimination of glandular secretions and other body toxins. The toes have meridian points for the eyes and sinuses. The bottom of the heel has a meridian point for the anus. The spinal column has meridian points along the inside edge of either foot.

Like the hands, the reflective points for the left side of the body are on the left foot and vice versa. This includes the eyes, ears, sinus cavities, and reproductive system. The meridian points for the ovaries are found on the area directly behind the ankle bone. The left ovary zone is on the left foot, and the right ovary zone is on the right one. The same zone point on the inner ankle bone is for a man's

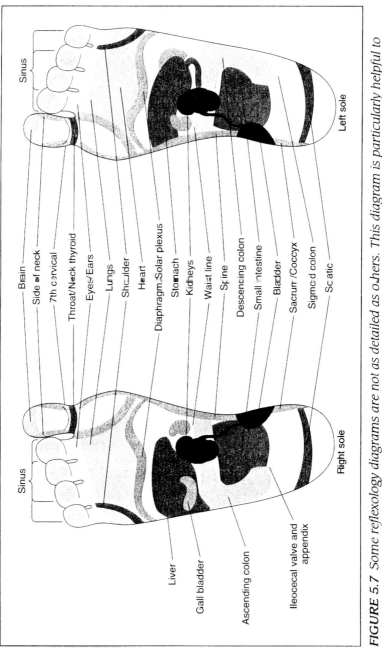

**FIGURE 5.7** *Some reflexology diagrams are not as detailed as others. This diagram is particularly helpful to show the pressure points on both feet that work the digestive tract.*

prostate and a woman's uterus. The Fallopian tubes are reflective on the meridians on the front of the foot, between the ankle bones.

### How to Engage the Points for Treatment

When you begin the session, you must establish confidence with clients so that they do not feel that you will tickle their feet when you touch them. Reflexology is not remotely connected to any tickling touch sensation. During the implementation phase, reflexology can actually be uncomfortable.

You may have some concern in dealing with a client's foot odor. Many people have strong, offensive foot smells. One method to combat this troublesome situation is to begin all reflexology exploratories with a mild cleansing of the feet. Pedicurists have the distinct advantage of being able to provide a pedicure before any reflexology session begins. The rest of us can wrap each of our client's feet in warm, wet towels that have been prescented with an aromatherapy essential oil. In addition, we can spray the feet with a mister filled with rosewater or any aromatherapy freshener. Wiping the feet with witch hazel also helps. Towel drying the feet and lightly powdering them will add enjoyment for everyone, client and reflexologist alike.

I begin the process by wrapping each foot in a dry, clean towel and placing a preheated electric foot bootie over the wrapped feet. Because heat is effective in increasing cellular activity and improving muscle relaxation, this allows the opportunity to perform a more effective reflexology treatment from the first appointment. This is, however, optional.

The standard method of beginning a reflexology exploratory is to start on the nondominant foot, that is, the right foot for left-handed people and vice versa. You grasp the entire foot between both of your hands. Because people store a great deal of pressure and stress in their ankles, your fingers begin at the base of the ankle, using a gentle twisting motion to rotate the foot and loosen the tension.

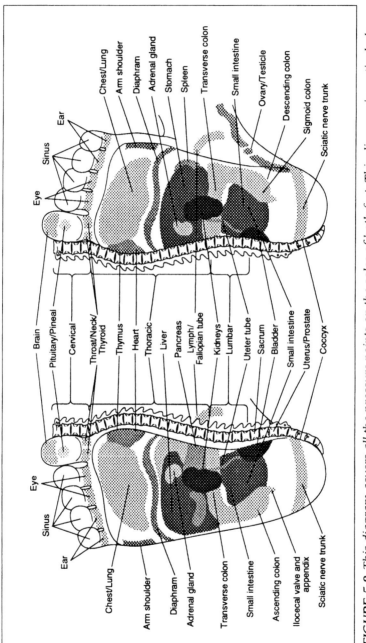

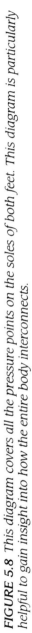

FIGURE 5.8 *This diagram covers all the pressure points on the soles of both feet. This diagram is particularly helpful to gain insight into how the entire body interconnects.*

Continue this twisting action all the way down to the toes. Then lift the sole of the foot forward to stretch the Achilles tendon. Now the foot is ready to be explored, using your thumb on your dominant hand as your guiding probe.

Because the entire body is reflective somewhere in the foot and ankle regions, I recommend that you begin with

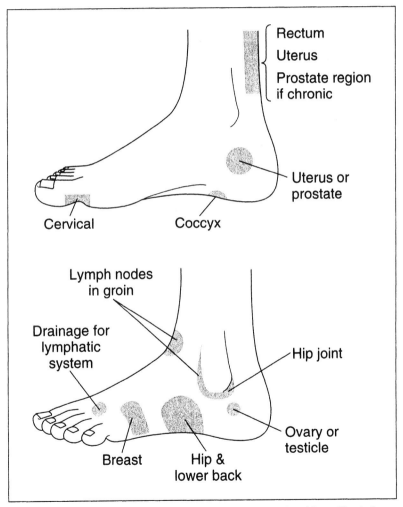

*FIGURE 5.9* Pressure points on the top, bottom, and ankles of both feet.

the toes, exploring each toe and working downward to the heel. Complete the exploratory on each foot separately.

Often a pattern will develop that will aid you in the implementation phase of the session. Be sure to take good notes as you conduct the exploratory. Record every meridian point that feels tender when you press on it. Which have crystal clusters underneath the meridian point? You will be developing a relationship with this client, and it will be important to keep accurate records. No one is expected to remember every detail of each client without keeping updated files.

## *Summary*

With a great deal of practice, you will become comfortable with all the various meridian points throughout the body. You will be able to evaluate the stress messages found throughout a client's body zones and give the necessary assistance. It is common to feel uncertain in the beginning. Remember that my mentor had me work the exploratory phase of the process every day for a year. Although she let me record what I thought would be the implementation process, she actually performed every one of them before I was allowed to do so.

The more seriously you take your studies, the more seriously your clients will take your work. The process is long, and I understand the frustrations of gaining expertise; however, the results and rewards are worth the trouble. If it were such an easy technique to master, there would be reflexology centers in every strip mall across the country. As of the writing of this book, I know of only one other master reflexologist in Southern California. Lynn Nelson and I have a great deal of respect for each other's work, and we are 180 miles from each other. In doing the research for this book, I made a wholehearted effort to find other well-trained reflexologists in my industry. I used the Yellow Pages as a guide to begin my search and then I just put the word out through various channels of communication. I did find 6 holistic health practitioners who offered reflexology in their practices. Five came from the Pacific Rim area, coming to America after decades of providing reflexology services in their homelands. Like my own mentor, they took years to perfect their skills.

# Chapter Six

## SPECIFIC AREAS OF CONCENTRATION

## Overview

The "magic" of reflexology is its ability to cover so many parts of the body from the soft organs to the skeletal system. Because you are not medically trained, only the conditions typical of everyday stresses and strains are included.

## Introduction

The joy of reflexology lies in its ability to aid so many different conditions. Although it is not common for a single session to bring complete relief from most problems, it will start the process along. The following are specific ailments that plague the average client. These conditions were chosen because they do not cross into the medical or disease arena. I strongly believe that the reflexologists in the beauty industry should limit their treatments to nondisease ailments.

## Headaches

This condition is especially common. Clients and staff members come to you for relief. One of the best reasons to choose reflexology over taking aspirin or other tablet medication is that the drugs circulate in the entire bloodstream, which means they are medicating the whole body for relief of only the headache. In the case of aspirin and all the extra-strength versions, the stomach lining is directly attacked.

While working in a salon, I found that on Saturday mornings my reflexology therapy was in great demand from the staff members. Several had the habit of drinking in excess on Friday nights, beginning at **Happy Hour** and continuing through the evening until the establishment closed. They would arrive to work on Saturday morning with a full-blown **hangover**. These employees commonly had a full day booked with appointments. They would feel so dreadful that they would want the receptionist to call their customers and reschedule them. The salon owner was never very happy with this scenario.

I would be recruited to perform the reflexology treatment on them to get them through the day. I worked the reflexes for the headache, offered some rebalancing of the system, and contributed to the employees' improved outlook. My efforts had a direct and positive effect on the relationship between the salon owner and the employees, who then had a better rapport with their clients.

Clients do not want their appointments canceled at the last minute, particularly on a Saturday morning. In addition, the employees usually would then tell their clients that they had come to work with a hangover and that the reflexologist "fixed them right up." I always found that to be an unusual declaration. I did not think that they should announce their lack of self-control, but it increased my business referrals from the clients for the exact same treatment.

Another popular use of this treatment is for clients who have hard working schedules or working environments. They can be experiencing a stress ache from pressures at the office. They will benefit from coming in for a treatment during their lunch break. Treatment can readjust their entire attitude about going back to work. This also works well if the clients come in for a session at the end of the work day. They go home in better condition and in a better mood than they would otherwise.

I had one client who had a very difficult job that put her in constant "stress ache of the head." Her fiancé wanted her to quit her job because he felt that he made enough money for both of them. However, she loved her work, even with the stress aches. She could not go home and expect to receive compassion from her fiancé when she had a headache. So she enjoyed coming in at the end of the day and getting a treatment when the stress ache was particularly strong. Then she was able to go home in a terrific mood. She and her fiancé benefited from this solution to her problem.

This particular treatment gains many referrals because the client is apt to talk about it to everyone. There is no stigma attached to speaking about a headache. It is not a condition that generates a feeling of "private information." Conditions such as depression or reproduction stress could be thought of as private matters, but not a headache.

When clients come in for a session, they often have not been touched in a caring way for a long time. The actual implementation of the session offers them a form of caress that they are lacking in their lives. This builds a great rapport between the reflexologist and the client.

You can choose meridian points on the ears, hands, or feet to offer relief. Depending on your particular professional title, you can select the part that best fits your other contact with your customer.

## On the Ear

There are two points at the top of the outer ear. One point is for the headache that is felt in front of the forehead and eye area. The second point is for the headache that seems to send pain to the back of the head.

Ask the client if the headache is felt more on the left side, perhaps behind the left eye or at the left temple. That would direct your treatment to begin on the left ear. The points are at the exact same spot on either ear. Place your thumb pad on the top, front side of the ear, where the curve

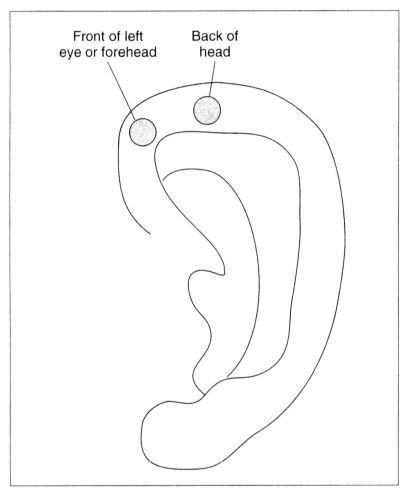

**FIGURE 6.1** *Pressure points on the left ear for treating headaches. (Points are the same for both ears.)*

of the ear begins to curl. Next, place your first finger pad on the back side of the exact point. Press gently but firmly on the point. Hold for the count of 3. Release your pressure and following a clockwise circular pattern massage that point to the count of 4. Stop and replace the firm pressure on the point. Hold for the count of 3. Then begin the massage movement in a counter-clockwise pattern to the count of 4. Repeat these steps twice. Release the ear from your fingers. Your client should be able to sense a reduction in the headache pain. The complete sensation should take between 5 and 10 minutes to go away. It is advisable to work both ears. Repeat the exact same procedure on the meridian points on the right ear.

You can repeat this procedure several times. If the client has a history of chronic headaches, you will need to work on this client several times. At first, it will be necessary to see your client 3 times a day for 5 days. You are readjusting the pattern of the pressure that has been building up in the client's head for a long time. This may seem like a lot of time and scheduling the appointments may be troublesome at first, but the results are always worth it in the end.

## On the Hand

Ask the client if the headache is felt more on the left side, perhaps behind the left eye or at the left temple. That would direct your treatment to begin on the left hand. The points are at the exact same spot on either hand. Each fingertip is part of the meridian point that reflects the head.

The base of each finger reflects the eyes and sinuses. Even the fleshy part of the thumb pad reflects the head. One point that is not easily explained is the center of the web tissue between the thumb and the index finger. It is a wonderful point to release intensive headaches caused by stress. The head is reflected in the tops of the fingers and the base of the fingers represent the lower sections of the neck and throat. The confusion comes with the soft tissue that connects the thumb and the index finger. There is a strong nerve cell that lies in the center of this web tissue that can release the pressures of a normal headache. Ancient writings referred to this area as the "third eye."

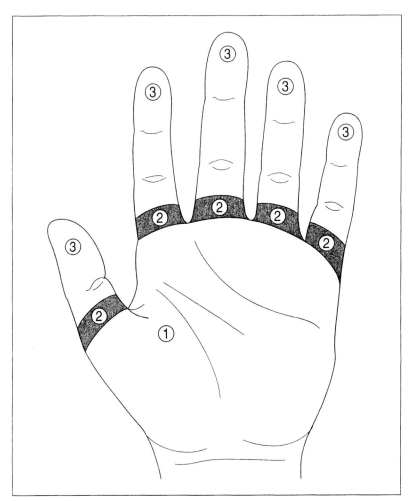

**FIGURE 6.2** *Pressure points on the left hand for treating headaches. 1, web; 2, left eye/left sinus; 3, head. (For right hand, use right eye/ right sinus.)*

Place your thumb on the top of the web tissue and your index finger on the palm side to complete the cycle. Press your thumb toward your index finger, trying to get them to touch; of course, that is not possible. The pressure you use is strong. Hold the point to the count of 5, releasing the intense pressure, but not moving off the point. Repeat this technique 3 or 4 times.

### On the Foot

The top of the big toe on both feet reflects the head. The base of each toe reflects the eyes and sinuses. The left and right are according to each side of the body also. Ask the client which side of the body had the pain sensation and begin your treatment on that side.

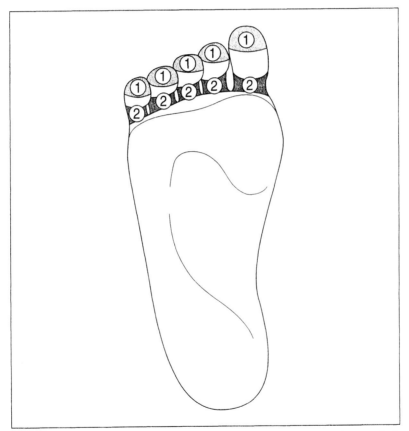

**FIGURE 6.3** *Pressure points on the foot for treating headaches. 1, left side of the head; 2, left eye/left sinus. (For right foot, use right side of head, right eye/right sinus.)*

When you begin, zone the meridian point on the top of each toe. Pressing firmly, and pumping gently, use the opposite hand's index finger for support of the toe when you apply direct pressure on the zone point. Repeat the pressing pumping action 3 times on each toe. Then move onto the base of each toe. Instead of finding a meridian point and applying direct pressure, roll the base of your client's toes between your thumb pad and your index finger. Make small pressurized circles over each individual toe. Do all the toes on each foot.

Then use your thumb pad again and press on each meridian on the top of each toe that corresponds to the head. Finally, place your thumb on the center of the fleshy part of the big toe and press very firmly for a count of 5. Release the pressure, but do not move off the meridian. Repeat the pressure hold 3 times.

### Client Profile

Sally Jones came in to the salon late in the day for her normal monthly facial, manicure, and pedicure. At the salon this is a package deal for a "Mini-Day of Beauty." The first service is the facial. While she was on the facial bed, she mentioned that she had a headache.

After we asked several key questions, we determined that the ache was over her left eye and brow. She did not have it when she woke up that morning. In fact, it only developed during a highly volatile company meeting. I decided to offer a quick reflexology "pressuring" (a term I made up to describe a short session, designed to work on a singular meridian area). I began the reflexology session with her left ear. I worked all the points. During the masking process, I asked Sally if the headache had lessened or resolved itself. She indicated that it was almost all gone. I then used her left hand and manipulated the meridian points there. I worked the points for less than 3 minutes.

I told the manicurist about Sally's headache, just in case she decided to offer more reflexology during her manicure or pedicure. (In this situation, it was not needed. Working her hand during the masking process eliminated the headache.)

## Backaches

It is important to ask the client if the back problems are generated from severe injuries, from a disease (e.g., spinal meningitis), or from daily stress or sitting too long in one position. You can handle the latter two conditions without getting into legal trouble. Be quick to suggest medical attention should you feel the situation warrants it.

This session is also extremely popular. Clients talk about the results with friends and family. The direct benefit for the reflexologist is the referrals this builds. The common nontrauma backache is a malady most people experience at some time. Knowing that they can go to you for comfort and release of the pressure is very reassuring.

More people are seated in front of computer terminals than ever before. This creates pressure in the spinal cord, particularly in their upper back, shoulder, and neck area. Whether a corporate executive or a college student, people find themselves forcing pressure against their vertebrae. In addition, heavy schedules during the work week force people to cram too much into their weekends. They can have a schedule of cleaning, washing the car, watching their children play sports, shopping, gardening, and socializing in the evening. Their backs are sure to take a direct hit from these events. By Monday or Tuesday, they cannot wait to see you!

There has been an increase in **infomercials** selling at-home fitness workout equipment directly to the consumer. More people have backaches and strains after using the machines and apparatus without the professional assistance they would find in a gym or exercise club. The reflexologist who is also a licensed masseuse or masseur could advise the client on the proper way to work the back muscles. Other reflexologists should refer their clients to either a licensed masseuse/masseur for advice or suggest that they consult with a physical fitness expert before continuing their workout at home. The reflexologist can provide assistance to the meridian points that are under attack, but the muscle aches must be worked out with a licensed masseuse/masseur.

At the salon, I offered a special "Weekend Unwinder" session for one half-hour appointment. The receptionist found it easy to suggest this service when booking other clients for appointments. Once it was known throughout the salon, it became a favorite among the single-parent family clients. They would book for this session at the beginning of a week that they knew ahead of time was going to be particularly hectic.

> **CAUTION:** It is important to note that if the client is experiencing back pain due to an accident or specific trauma, it is **not** recommended that you attempt to offer reflexology as a solution to this kind of spinal/backache.

The following discussion pertains to clients with mild backache and back soreness.

### On the Ear

The outer edges of the ears "reflect" the client's spinal column. For this condition, you determine which ear to manipulate by which is the dominant side of the client. Begin your treatment with the left ear for a right-handed person and vice versa.

Roll the outer edge of the ear between your thumb and your first finger, starting at the base of the earlobe and working upward to the top of the ear. Your finger pressure

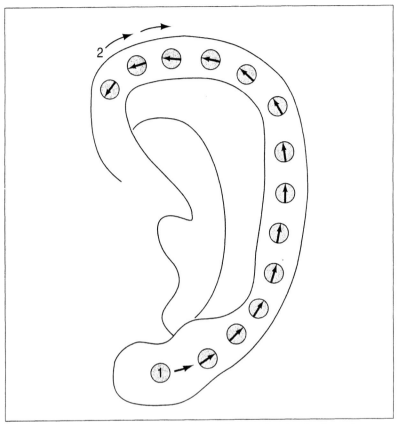

*FIGURE 6.4 Pressure points on the ear for treating backaches. Step one moves up the ear; step two moves down the ear.*

should be firm and your movements smooth. This is one reflexology treatment that flows similar to a regular massage movement. Then reverse your direction. It is a good practice to work all the meridian points reflecting the spinal column. Therefore repeat this procedure twice on both ears.

## On the Hand

The outer edge of both thumbs along with the base of each hand reflect the entire skeletal column from the top of the neck to the base of the spine through to the area called the "tail bone" or **coccyx**. Work on the client's nondominant hand first. Using your thumb, manipulate the meridian points on the thumb and base of the hand de-

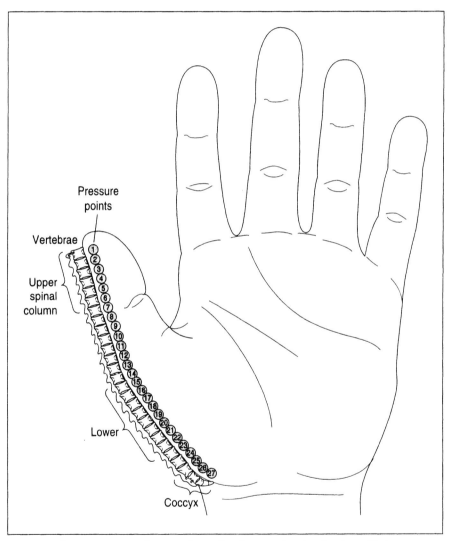

**FIGURE 6.5** *Pressure points on the palm for treating backaches. (Points are the same for the right hand.)*

pending on where the soreness is on the client's back. Upper backache is on the upper part of the outer edge of the thumb. Lower back pain is reflective on the lower edge of the thumb and base of the hand. Look at the drawing for clarification of the points.

Use very firm pressure, working slowly over the designated area. Each point is pressed independently. Your thumb moves along the edge of the thumb, as if there were vertebrae one after the other along the edge. (Refer to the drawing.) Repeat the firm, slow pressure 4 times. Work down the thumb and base and then reverse direction and work upward. Manipulate meridians on both hands.

### On the Foot

Similar to the outer edge of the thumbs, the entire skeletal column is reflective along the outer edges of the big toe and along the instep and heel. The meridian points are the same on the left and right foot.

Manipulate the right foot for a left-handed person and vice versa. Ask your client where the pain is located—upper, middle, or lower back. The meridian points begin for the head and neck on the big toe's outer edge; the middle of the back is in the instep and the lower back follows along the top of the heel. The coccyx is at the base of the heel.

Use your thumb pad and manipulate each meridian independently. Work your thumb downward, using slow, firm pressure. Then reverse direction. Repeat this pressure motion 5 times.

### Client Profiles

Harry Smith came into the salon for a haircut. As he checked in at the front desk, he mentioned that he had slept the night before on the sofa and now his back was sore. The receptionist passed along this information to his stylist's assistant, who took the initiative to offer some reflexology to help his backache. She quickly explained that she would

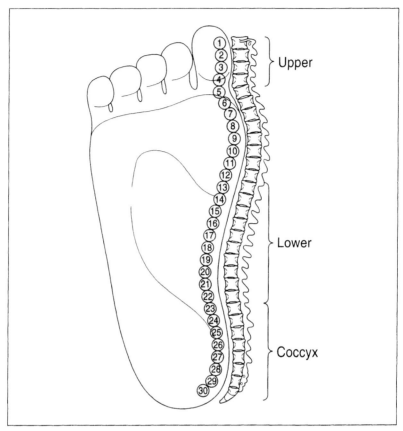

**FIGURE 6.6** *Pressure points on the right foot for treating backaches. (Points are the same for the left foot.)*

apply some firm but gentle pressure on his ears while he was at the shampoo bowl. She asked Harry whether he is right- or left-handed. He answered that he is left-handed. So she began manipulating the meridian points on the outer edge of his left ear. Then she worked on the right ear. Harry was not aware of any immediate change in his back, but he said the reflexology felt great and gave her a large tip. He mentioned to the stylist how pleased he was with the assistant's attention. The stylist suggested to Harry that he get a full reflexology foot treatment with the manicurist. Harry immediately agreed, and the appointment was set up to be completed after his haircut. This is the way a salon can gain a reputation for quality service and make more money for the salon and its employees. Harry Smith can now become a multiservice client. The more services customers receive while in the salon, the more loyal clients they become.

Janet Coe was scheduled for a pedicure. When she arrived, she requested a manicure too because she just moved into a new apartment and while loading and unloading all of her cartons, she ruined her nails. Her manicurist was totally booked and could not fit in an unscheduled manicure; however, another manicurist was able to do one after she finished with the pedicure. This worked out well; Janet's toes could dry while she had her nails done. While she was in the pedicure bath soaking her feet, she mentioned how sore her back was after all the lifting and moving she had done. Her manicurist told her that she would perform some extra reflexology manipulations for her spinal column while doing her pedicure. She was given a reflexology exploratory and then a full implementation session. Janet loved the treatment. By the time she was ready for her manicure 90 minutes later, she commented on how wonderful she felt. Her back did not hurt any more. Her manicurist recommended that Janet come in a few days to get an overall balancing reflexology session. Janet booked it as she left the salon.

## Digestion Troubles

In today's society, people are rushed throughout the day. Making time to relax and eat slowly is often difficult. Fast food is making it impossible to think about slowing down the time it takes to eat. This forces the stomach to digest partially chewed food in an atmosphere of time constraints and physical and emotional stress. In addition to bad eating habits, our clients are often growing older, which makes their metabolism slow down and be less efficient. The end result of all of these factors is an increase in heartburn and stomachaches. Advising your clients to change the way they eat, how they prepare the food, and the amount of time set aside to consume it would all help reduce the digestion problems plaguing so many people.

Reflexology can assist a client in two areas. First is the relief of minor stomachaches caused by simple daily stress or bad eating habits. The treatment technique described in the following paragraphs addresses those situations. Another benefit of reflexology is the tracking of an **ulcer**. There will be crystal clusters in the meridian points relating to the stomach when an ulcer is developing. Even when you destroy the clusters, the client will need medical attention.

> **CAUTION:** Ulcers are a serious medical problem that should not be ignored. The two most common kinds of ulcers are the **peptic ulcer** and the **duodenal ulcer** in the upper portion of the small intestine. The duodendum lies right next to the stomach. The powerful stomach acids seep into the lining of the duodendum, causing the ulcers to form.

Always suggest to your clients that they consult with their physicians regarding any stomach ailments. Once they are under a doctor's care, you can offer reflexology sessions as part of the treatment to reduce their discomfort.

Although we are not medical practitioners, our reflexology exploratory phase can alert clients that trouble is developing and direct them in the proper medical direction. In this situation, reflexology becomes an effective preventive treatment so an ulcer does not progress to requiring surgery.

Other stomachaches are created from the previously mentioned life-style choices. Although they are not serious, that does not diminish the discomfort surrounding them. Here the reflexologist can provide immediate release of the discomfort.

You must understand that the digestive system is made up of several parts, the stomach and intestines being significant members. The gallbladder, liver, pancreas, and colon all play a role in the processing of food. The entire process begins with the intake of food through the mouth. It is swallowed and travels down the **pharynx** and **esophagus** before it arrives in the stomach. To properly treat the problem, the entire system would have to be worked on. This would require the reflexologist to begin the treatment session with the meridian reflex points for the:

- mouth
- pharynx
- esophagus
- stomach
- small and large intestines
- ileocecal valve
- four parts of the colon: **transverse**, ascending, **descending**, and **sigmoid**
- anus

This poses a special problem for the reflexologist in the beauty business. Within our beauty licensing, it is out of bounds to work the entire system. We would need a medical practitioner to guide us. In the salon, spa, and full-service beauty business, we cannot use reflexology to successfully reduce all the discomfort and pain associated with digestion problems. For various reasons, it is best for the beauty industry reflexologist to work only on the lower elements of the digestive system.

First is the fact that by manipulating the four parts of the colon and anus meridian, release of fecal matter is possible. Second, it eliminates the possibility that the client will misinterpret the nonmedical approach and get the reflexologist in a legal confrontation. Third, working the lower portion of the digestive tract will release trapped **flatulence** (gas). Fourth, particularly for the beginner, it is best to keep the treatment routines simple.

Some digestive troubles arise as normal responses to events going on inside the client's body. One common digestive situation occurs during pregnancy. First is morning sickness that often afflicts the expectant mother. The resulting nausea makes eating an unpleasant experience. Second, as the baby grows and the body expands to accommodate this growth, the baby forces pressure to build on the internal organs. The woman can struggle with stomach problems for several months. Third is the development of **hemorrhoids**. The pressure of the baby on the lower organs causes these blood sacs to form around the anus. As the pregnancy goes to term, hemorrhoids are annoying. Although they do not normally pose a serious health risk, they can be directly associated as a cause of **anemia**. Hemorrhoids are also physically uncomfortable. The natural healing methods of the body will attempt to correct the condition. Reflexology can help the body do so more quickly. The client will be very grateful for this assistance.

The reflexologist quickly becomes her new "best friend." The pregnant woman cannot take medications without subjecting her baby to their effects. Therefore, selecting reflexology as a source of relief is the perfect answer. The reflexologist can also help young fathers who experience "**sympathy pains**."

Other sources of digestive problems include the flu or those arising after minor surgery requiring **sodium pentothal** and after some dental procedures such as teeth extractions. Reflexology can provide assistance in reducing the indigestion brought on by these conditions although running to the reflexologist for these situations is highly unlikely as well as impractical. A better alternative would be to teach your clients a few tips on hand manipulation so that they can render assistance to themselves.

Do not be concerned about turning away business. This will actually have the opposite effect. The clients will appreciate your kindness in looking out for their better health and come in for more complete sessions.

## On the Hand

The stomach's meridian points are on the left hand, in the center of the palm. There is not just a singular spot the size of a dot to look for. As you begin learning how to work with reflexology, you will get accustomed to finding this area. The chart will help to locate it. Using your dominate hand's thumb, locate the center of the meridian point area.

Begin by moving in small circles in a counter-clockwise motion over the center area of the meridian points. Make 3 small circles. Stop and place direct pressure on the center meridian with your thumb pad. Repeat the small circles for 3 rotations in a clockwise pattern.

## On the Foot

The stomach's meridian points are on the left foot. The area is on the outside section of the instep. Just as on the hand, there is not just a singular dot to look for. Look at the chart for help in locating it. Using your dominant hand's thumb, locate the center of the meridian point area. Begin by moving in small circles in a counter-clockwise motion over the center area of the meridian points. Make 3 small circles. Stop and place direct pressure on the center meridian with your thumb pad. Then repeat the small circles for 3 rotations in a clockwise pattern. The foot is much stronger in getting reflexology to respond to the inner body. It is possible to bring relief quickly to a client with stomach cramps.

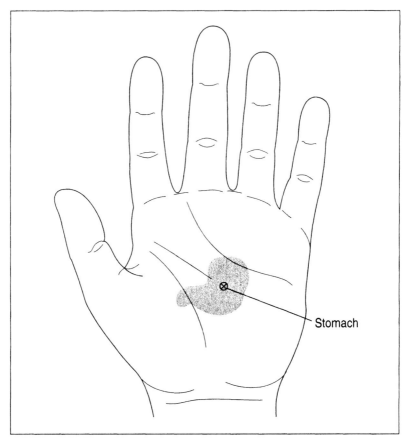

*FIGURE 6.7* Pressure point area on the palm for treating digestion problems. (Points are the same for the right palm.)

## Client Profile

Depending on the amount of privacy available for the relief of the client's discomfort, the hand meridians are the best choice. You can manipulate the points in a matter of moments. Do not forget that most digestive troubles will include a buildup of flatuence. I have found it best to bring up this obvious factor in a jovial manner. The client will begin to "pass wind" quickly. It can even begin during the treatment. (Most often this will happen.) You do not want

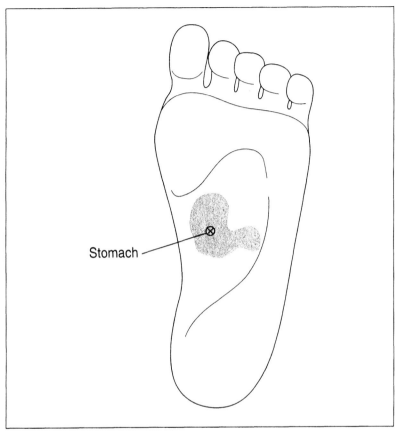

**FIGURE 6.8** *Pressure point area on the foot for treating digestion problems. (Points are the same for the right foot.)*

to add to your client's discomfort by making the person feel embarrassed. Try to find a secluded place in your business that will offer a feeling of privacy, but preferably with adequate ventilation.

Working the feet would be a wise choice if you can allow the client to recline on a facial bed or massage table. If the client is just sitting in a chair, having to raise the feet to work on them can put additional pressure on the lower stomach and intestines.

### A Day Spa Business Profile

When a brand new day spa opened, the owners wanted an opportunity to do joint ventures with other businesses in their immediate area. This would help them to connect with the other small business owners and spread the word that they exist. The spa manager consulted with me and we came up with the following program.

The idea was to offer the reflexology sessions to customers of the other businesses. The other businesses would benefit in two direct ways. First, their employees were offered a complimentary reflexology session to be able to say that they had experienced one and let their clients know what they liked about it. Second, they were given promotional material that had certificates for $5 and $10 off the half-hour and full-hour sessions that would only be available for their clients. Their clients were happy to receive the special discount certificates.

On review of the neighboring businesses, we decided that the fitness center and 3 weight loss centers would be good target markets for the reflexology sessions on digestion. Clients of both kinds of businesses would have personal reasons to be changing their eating habits. When people change their eating style, their digestive process is affected too.

The spa manager presented the idea to the other owners. They all agreed to try it, and the endeavor was a huge success.

## Reproduction System Problems

### Men

Reflexology can assist men in determining if any difficulty is developing in the **prostate**. If prostate cancer runs in their family medical history, this is particularly important. In addition, most men do not seek out medical examinations, particularly for this gland. Most men would rather have a reflexology meridian point be checked than go to a proctologist for an annual examination. Obviously, if there is a real problem, only a doctor can help.

Early detection is important to discover prostate problems before they become more serious. An effective reflexology exploratory phase will not uncover a crystal cluster in the meridian point. The meridian point for the prostate is on the inner ankle bone. It will feel very tender and spongelike on the meridian point. It will be very, very uncomfortable. This will alert the client to seek medical attention to further explore the possibility that trouble in the prostate exists.

Do not be an alarmist! No man wants to hear news that he may have a problem in his prostate. Carefully inquire if he is currently having difficulty with urinating, or experiencing tenderness during masturbation or intercourse. Ask if he has a known family history of prostate cancer. If the man is under age 50, it is probably due to reasons other than a disease. Overactivity or underactivity will cause sensitivity in the prostate. Reflexology would send a wrong message. When in doubt, the less said, the better.

## Women

Reflexology cannot assist a woman who has problems with conception although other books suggest the contrary. My personal trainer had never seen it happen and neither have I.

Women go to the doctor much more regularly than men. Because women have a regular menstrual cycle, they are constantly aware of their internal organs. Reflexology can provide help in several different ways—removing menstrual cramps, determining when the ovulation cycle begins, and checking to see if pregnancy has occurred. For women who are approaching menopause, reflexology can track the activity schedule of their ovaries, which will help them determine when the cycle is ready to stop.

The meridian points for the **ovaries** are found on the area directly behind the ankle bone. The left ovary zone is on the left foot, and the right ovary zone is on the right foot. The same zone point on the inner ankle bone is for a man's prostate and a woman's **uterus**. The **Fallopian tubes** are reflective on the meridians on the front of the foot, between the ankle bones. These meridian points are extremely sensitive! Even light pressure can send strong sensations of discomfort to the client. During the exploratory, you must be careful and take excellent notes on exactly what you feel on each meridian.

If a problem is developing, you will feel crystal cluster deposits on other meridian points on the soles of the feet, but not on the reproduction points. They will feel tender and have a spongy sensation under your fingers. During the implementation phase, you will be pumping the points, not crushing crystals.

During the exploratory phase, use your dominant thumb and index finger. Place your thumb on the outside part of the area behind the client's ankle bone and the index finger on the inside part. Try to press both fingers together; if the tissue between your fingers feels like a small marshmallow is stuck there, the body is sending a message about the ovaries.

One meridian point for the ovary will be spongy and the other flat when **ovulation** occurs. As long as a woman has both of her ovaries intact, usually they alternate releasing the egg each month. Both meridian points will be spongy when she is pregnant. If one side is constantly spongy, one ovary is working all the time and the other is not, which will happen during the early stages of menopause. Suggest that the client seek her gynecologist's opinion. Be sure that you are not mistaken as offering medical advice.

## Pregnancy

This is the most important event in a woman's life. It is filled with wonderment and worry. For the first-time pregnant woman the experience is filled with questions, some of which have difficult answers. But the query "Can a reflexologist help make it an easier pregnancy?" is an easy one to answer—yes, absolutely, positively yes! The reflexologist will make an easy pregnancy even more comfortable and a difficult pregnancy less traumatic.

**NOTE:** The author is not saying that reflexology makes a difficult pregnancy easy.

With the woman's body going through so many changes, the meridian points/reflexes are put on high alert. Everything on and in the body is more noticeable.

**EXAMPLE:** If a client has a regular problem with flatulence under normal conditions, during her pregnancy it is drastically more intense.

Special indigestion problems can occur during pregnancy (refer to section on Digestion Troubles, page 81). Morning sickness can make eating an unpleasant experience. As the baby grows and the body expands, the baby increases pressure on the stomach, intestines, and **diaphragm**. The expectant mother can struggle with stomach problems for several months, during which time she cannot take medications. In addition, a pregnant woman's feet will often swell and bloat. She frequently feels she needs extra attention. Her mood swings can be particularly strong.

Selecting reflexology as a source of relief is the perfect answer. During the treatment session, an overall balancing will also be in order.

The reflexologist offers a sense of caring, an element of specialized attention, and treatment sessions to ease some of the normal nuisances of pregnancy. Mild depression, swollen hands and feet, constipation, intestinal distress, headaches, backaches, and nausea can all be aided while being perfectly safe for the baby.

Use the woman's hands or feet, although most often she will more appreciate the service on her feet. You can do more than one specialty, depending on what is bothering her at the time. During the 9 months, certain ailments and conditions will become more prevalent.

> **EXAMPLE:** Through the first trimester, morning sickness may dominate, and through the last trimester she may have more problems with her bladder and bowels. Adjust your sessions accordingly.

For the client with sufficient financial resources, bimonthly visits would be ideal until the eighth month, when weekly visits are beneficial to relax and de-stress the pregnant client. Have less financially secure women come in as often as possible. Perhaps as a baby shower gift, such a woman could be given a gift certificate for a series of sessions with you. If a group of coworkers or relatives contributed, the gift would be reasonably priced and the client would greatly benefit from it.

At the salon where I worked, I posted a list of special gift ideas for wedding showers, baby showers, and wedding presents for the couple. The series of reflexology sessions was a popular choice. Treatment selections can be an individual session or a blend of several as part of the routine, including backache, constipation, depression, headache, and overall balance. Review all the diagrams for each of these conditions. You can combine several in one session. All of these can be done while the pregnant client is moderately reclining on a facial bed that has the back raised. Do not have her lie flat on her back.

## Premenstrual Syndrome

Premenstrual syndrome (PMS) was misunderstood by doctors and the general public for centuries. Because of this misunderstanding, women from all walks of life were branded "the period bitch," "the menstrual maniac," and many other unattractive names. Not all women experience the pain, emotional swings, and overall reduction of self-esteem during the time between ovulation and the actual blood flow of their menses.

Certain patterns now help us determine when the PMS attacks will occur. Hormone surges are a major cause of the problem. Women will often complain of tenderness in their breasts. Headaches are often a side effect. Suggest that they reduce their intake of caffeine and salt.

Researchers have discovered that women who have only one working ovary will be more likely to experience the negative effects of the overworked ovary. It does not have the ability to shut down every other cycle as does a system with two normally functioning ovaries. The intensity of the flow is heavier and lasts longer. In addition, a woman can have both of her ovaries intact and working; however, one side will be more responsive to all the hormone rushes that fill the body during the menses. For women who fall into this classification, knowing which ovary causes the PMS symptoms is beneficial information.

The reflexologist can offer her this information. By tracking the meridian points for both ovaries and Fallopian tubes and uterus, you will be able to judge which side is the more sensitive. Giving this information to the client allows her the freedom to work her schedule around the event.

The meridian points on the feet and hands for the ovaries, Fallopian tubes, and uterus will reveal what is going on with these three important parts of the reproduction cycle. If a woman could know in advance what is going on inside her body as she goes through her menses each month, she could plan her hectic schedules to reduce her external stress while her biologic clock is increasing her internal stress. You can give this information to your client by having her come in for a 60-second review of these meridians once a week for 2 months. The average cycle is really 6 weeks long. Even though the menses occurs every 28 to 32 days, there are several days before and after the cycle that are important to track. Because the client will start this 60-second review at any given point that is convenient to the two of you, her menses cycle is hard to pinpoint during the first few sessions. That is why you use the 8-week evaluation time chart when you begin the review.

You chart the degree of sensitivity response to these meridian points. These 3 areas will feel spongy and swollen to the finger. The client will say that these areas are tender to the touch. You should note on the record:

- When she does have her period
- How long it lasts
- What effects she had during the period

For many women PMS is a serious issue because it can destroy their emotional outlook for several days, sometimes longer. Helping a client cope with these strong mood swings and body aches will be very much appreciated.

**EXAMPLE:** Client A finds out after 3 months of tracking that her left ovary triggers the PMS attacks. Through her reflexologist, she learns which month the left side is active. Now she can plan her busy schedule to allow more relaxation time when her left ovary releases the egg. Once she is aware when she will be more receptive to the mood swings and the physical discomfort accompanying PMS, she can plan to do things to reduce them. Being prepared for an unpleasant time will not make the event go away. It will make it more tolerable for everyone involved. This includes her partner, her children, family members, and her coworkers.

## On the Hand

To reduce stress associated with PMS, you will need to work all the points for the entire reproduction system, the

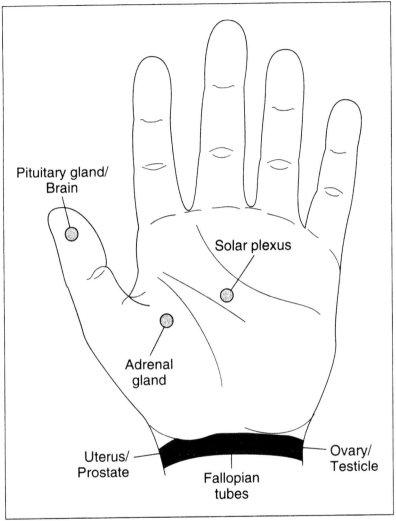

*FIGURE 6.9 Pressure points on the palm for treating stress associated with premenstrual syndrome. (Points are the same for the right hand.)*

meridians for the **solar plexus**, **adrenal gland**, **pituitary gland**, and the brain. Check the chart for the locations of the meridian points. The solar plexus is on both hands, at the center of the palm. The adrenal gland point is on both hands, at the fleshy part below the thumb. The point for the pituitary gland and brain is the same and is on the fleshy part of the thumb.

Use your dominant thumb and use pressing and pumping motions on all of these points. Do the complete rotations 4 times. Work the ovary points, then the uterus and Fallopian tube meridian points, followed by the solar plexus, adrenal gland, and finally the pituitary and brain points.

### On the Foot

The same points on the hands will be duplicated on the feet. They are even more responsive on the feet. The solar plexus is on both feet, at the lower edge of the balls of the feet. The adrenal gland is on both feet, at the top section of the instep, on the inside edge. The point for the pituitary gland and brain is the same and is on both feet on the fleshy part of the big toes.

Use your dominant thumb and use pressing and pumping motions on all of these points. Do the complete rotations 4 times. Work the ovary points, then the uterus and Fallopian tube meridian points, followed by the solar plexus, adrenal gland, and finally the pituitary and brain points.

### Client Profile

In dealing with PMS, one of the nicest elements of reflexology is the ability to determine which ovary is causing the symptoms. By knowing it ahead of time, the client can work around it and plan her activities accordingly.

Karen is a good example. She felt her life was out of control because of how crazy things became when she had PMS. Karen would tell me that her family would make excuses to stay away from her during a PMS attack. She totally understood their reactions, but unfortunately she couldn't run away from herself! This left her very upset.

We were able to keep track of the internal releases of hormones throughout her system through reflexology

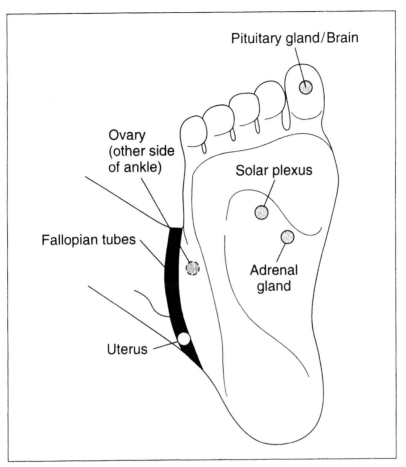

*FIGURE 6.10 Pressure points on the foot for treating stress associated with premenstrual syndrome. (Points are the same for the left foot.)*

exploratories of the 3 meridian points for the ovaries, Fallopian tubes, and uterus. Because she was coming in for the 60-second reviews, it was easy to determine which of the 3 parts of the reproduction system was causing the PMS symptoms. By charting the process, we determined that her PMS symptoms were brought on by one of her ovaries. Once we knew the pattern, we had a gauge to help us understand when the process would begin.

In Karen's case, her left ovary was the one that brought on the PMS. What was a bit unusual was that her left ovary would kick in twice as often as her right. After careful monitoring, we discovered that she would have the lightest period on the month that her right ovary released the egg. For two consecutive periods, she would experience PMS. Her period lasted longer on one of the left ovary cycles but not the other.

All the careful charting and evaluation allowed Karen the freedom to plan ahead. Together we were able to understand when a PMS attack was most likely to occur. Now she could plan lighter work loads and more relaxation time on the days PMS was due. She felt more in control of her life and that gave her a sense of accomplishment. It also made her easier to be around, which pleased her family!

## Menstrual Cramps

### On the Hand

The left hand reflects the left ovary and vice versa. Once you determine which ovary is causing the cramps, you work that meridian point. Place your dominant thumb on the outside edge of the base of the wrist. Apply gentle but firm pressure on the meridian, and then pump the point 4 times. Move your thumb on the other side of the base of the wrist and repeat the same procedure.

Then place your index finger along the top side of the wrist, as you slide your thumb along the base of the inside of the wrist. Slide your thumb back and forth 3 times. This is the meridian point for the Fallopian tube. It is not necessary to do both ovaries and Fallopian tubes, but it would not be damaging to do all the meridian points either. Working these meridians 48 hours before the client's ovulation

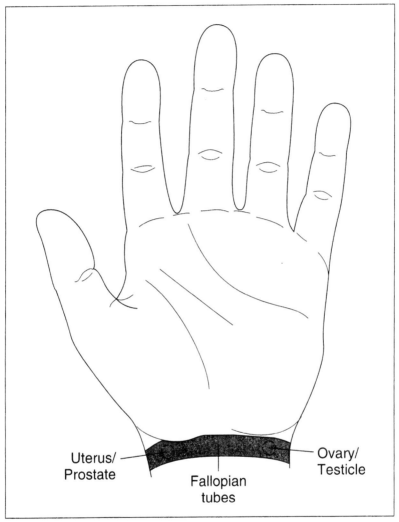

**FIGURE 6.11** *Pressure points on the palm for treating menstrual cramps. (Points are the same on right hand.)*

begins will help lessen the chance that any cramping will occur. The same is true for the 48-hour time frame before the menses begins.

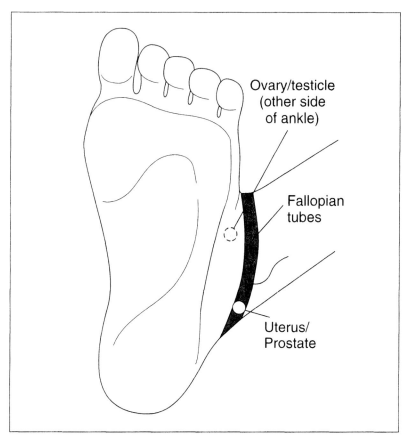

**FIGURE 6.12** *Pressure points on the ankle for treating menstrual cramps. (Points are the same on right ankle.)*

### On the Foot

This precautionary treatment is also effective on the feet. The left foot reflects the left side of the reproduction system and vice versa. The meridian for the uterus is on the right foot. Ask your client which side is cramping.

Place your dominant thumb on the outside space be-low the ankle of the corresponding side. Your index finger is on the inside space. Apply gentle but firm pressure on the meridian and then pump the point 4 times. Move your thumb on the top side of the area where the foot meets the leg and slide your thumb along this area. Slide your thumb back and forth 3 times. Gentle pressing and pumping are also required. It is not necessary to do both sides, but it cannot hurt the system if you do.

## Client Profile

Charlotte came to me through a referral by a friend who was a long-standing waxing client. During one of the waxing appointments for her friend, we discussed the power of reflexology to determine the activity level of the ovaries and reduce cramping. She then told Charlotte about our conversation.

Charlotte was having a tough time with menstrual cramps. The typical OTC medications made her stomach upset, forcing her to have cramps or nausea. The idea of a noninvasive treatment to rid her of cramps seemed too good to be true. She called the salon and asked many questions. I suggested that she come in for treatment. Because I had performed hundreds of sessions just for cramping, I was positive that reflexology would lessen her cramps. In fact, most often reflexology will relieve cramping.

When she arrived, I took a thorough evaluation, then began my exploratory on her nondominant hand and foot. I found out she had ovulated on her left side, which was her dominant side. Therefore, I performed the implementation phase on the left hand and foot. She came to her first session with cramps and left an hour later with a genuine smile. It worked! We then set her up on a regular treatment program. She was to return 24 to 48 hours before she ovulated. Charlotte became a wonderful promoter of my business. All of her female friends learned of my reflexology sessions and most of them came in for treatment.

# Sinus Problems

Many factors can create sinus inflammation. Heredity is one; if the parents have conditions that cause stress on the sinus sacs, they can pass on the tendency to their children. Allergies can be hereditary or just a weakness in one's own immune system. Bacteria and viruses also can irritate the sacs. Often the eyes, nose, and temples will be sensitive when the sinus sacs are inflamed. There are six sacs—2 under the eyebrows, 2 at the temples, and 2 under the eye sockets.

Medications have strong side effects. Pills can cause drowsiness and nasal sprays can be addictive. The body will build up a resistance to many medications. This forces the client to either increase the dosage or find stronger formulas to use to get the sinuses back to normal. Unfortunately, with the constant use of medications, the client's sinuses seldom return to normal. The medications will leave a trace of drug within the sinus cavity after the client stops taking it. A dependency slowly builds inside the sinus sac, causing the client to continue using the medications for longer periods of time. Reflexology can help relieve the pressure and aid the body's ability to drain the sinuses with zero side effects.

## On the Hand

To relieve the sinuses, other connected areas (eyes, throat, neck, and head) are important to manipulate. The meridian points for the sinuses and the eyes are the same zones. The base of each finger on the left hand reflects the sinus and eye on the left side of the body; the right hand works for the other. On either hand the bottom of the first digit and the base of the thumb have reflective meridians for the head, neck, and throat. Place your thumb on the meridian point, apply firm pressure, hold for the count of 5. Then pump the zone for the count of 3. Work each finger and thumb separately. Repeat this procedure 3 times.

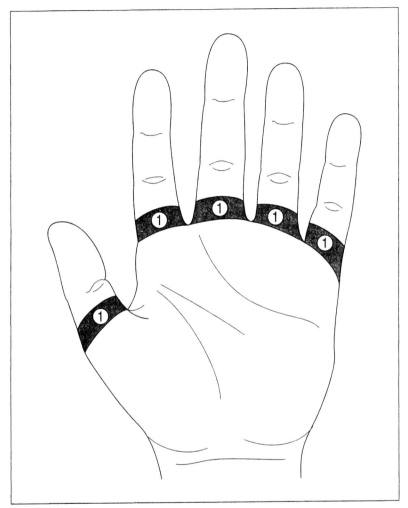

*FIGURE 6.13* *Pressure points on the palm for treating sinus problems. 1, sinus drains. (Points are the same on right hand.)*

## On the Foot

The eyes and sinus points are on the same zones on each toe, the base of the toe. The left foot reflects the left side of the body and vice versa. The throat and neck are at

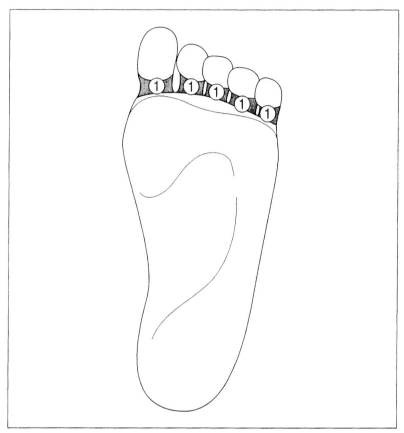

**FIGURE 6.14** *Pressure points on the foot for treating sinus problems. 1, sinus drains. (Points are the same on right foot.)*

the base of the big toes. Use your thumb on each meridian point individually. Place your thumb on the meridian point, apply firm pressure, and hold for the count of 5. Then pump the zone for the count of 3. Work each finger and thumb separately. Repeat this procedure 3 times.

## Client Profile

In my opinion, if the world knew how well reflexology works on relieving sinus pressure and releasing the fluid, we could eliminate the need for OTC sinus medications. Reflexology never has any absorbency problems, has no side-effects, and works better over time.

Carol and Cheryl had a lifelong struggle with their sinuses. They did have a predisposed hereditary weakness, which was the initial problem. Then they became addicted to using nasal sprays. Their systems became so dependent that they could not go a day without the spray. Then they came into the salon for a haircut and through conversation heard about reflexology treatments. They signed up immediately. Because they had been suffering with sinus problems for so long, they needed to have several sessions. It would take time to redirect their sinus patterns. We set them up on dual visits, so they could be together. Their appointments were 3 times a week for the first month. After the first month, they responded so well that their appointments were set to twice a week. By the third month, they needed to come in only once a week.

## Overall Balance

Sometimes clients do not have any one body area that is causing a problem. These clients just feel out of sorts, with no known reason to pinpoint the change. The classic "umbrella" rationale is stress.

We recognize good stress along with negative stress. When clients complain that they are just not feeling like themselves, with sleep patterns broken, they are coming to you for answers. For these clients, reflexology can bring balance back to their body. Working all the meridian points in either their hands or feet will accomplish this task. Using the charts, you can begin your session with the usual exploratory and then go into the implementation phase.

You can also use this treatment routine along with others to offer a more complete wellness program for the client. Depression, pregnancy, stress reduction, and indigestion are just some of the many conditions that would benefit by adding this routine to the manipulations for the specific conditions.

This is one of the most universal treatments available. It will blend with all of the other treatment segments or stand on its own merit. My trainer used to say, "Shelley, when you are uncertain where to begin your treatment series or segments, start with the 'overall balance' routine, and you will not fail to meet your client's needs. This one segment is the cornerstone to so many of the others." This was good advice for me and so I pass it along to you.

### On the Ear

Start at the very top of the outer edge of the ear all the way down to the earlobe. Use your thumbs and index fingers. Using both hands, and work both of the client's ears at the same time. Place your thumb on the inside of the rim and the index finger behind to support the pressure of the thumb. Slowly and firmly work all the meridian points, from the top of the ear to the end of the earlobe. Put pressure on each reflex point and hold the pressure to the count of 4. Move to the next point. Repeat this gentle firm pressure cycle over the entire ear. Check with the diagram for the location of each meridian point.

When you have completed the movement, stop and place your fingers over the ears to gently caress the entire ear for a holding pattern of 3 seconds. Lift your hands off the ears. Ask if the client feels more relaxed. If the answer is no, repeat the entire process.

### On the Hand

Start with the top of the body, by beginning with the fingertips on your client's nondominant hand. Using your thumb, manipulate the top portion of the client's thumb, which is the reflex point for the brain. The movement of your thumb is a pumping action. Work the meridian 3 times.

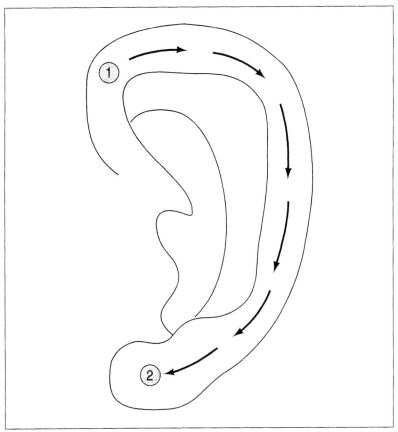

*FIGURE 6.15* *Pressure points on the ear for treating overall balance.*
*1, beginning point; 2, ending point.*

Then proceed to pump the tops of each finger separately. You are working the reflex points for the brain on each finger. Gentle but firm pressure should be used.

Next you need to work the reflex points for the spinal column. They run along the outer edge of the thumb, down along the base toward the wrist. These are the meridian points for the entire spinal column, a major center for stress to build when the body's inner balance is off. Move your thumb along the meridians by sliding down the outer edge

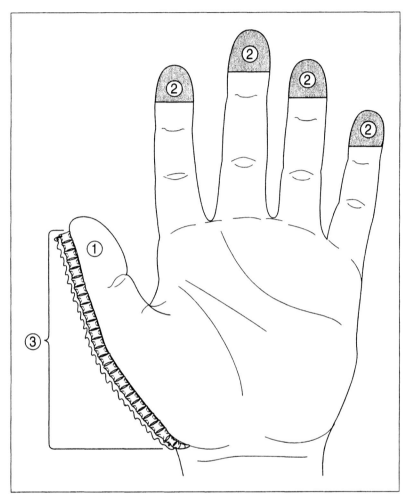

**FIGURE 6.16** *Pressure points on the palm for treating overall balance. 1, brain reflex; 2, brain reflex; 3, spinal reflex.*

of the client's thumb, very slowly. Then use tiny circles to work in an upward direction. Repeat the sliding down and circling back upward 3 or 4 times.

Repeat the entire process on the dominant hand. Ask if the client feels more at ease. If needed, repeat the entire process on both hands 2 or 3 times. Give the client's body at least 10 to 12 minutes to respond. Remember that reflexology is effective, but it does take time to get the relay to the brain and back again.

### On the Foot

The reflexes on the feet are the most powerful to regain inner balance. The meridian points for the head are on the tops of the toes. At the middle of the big toe is the

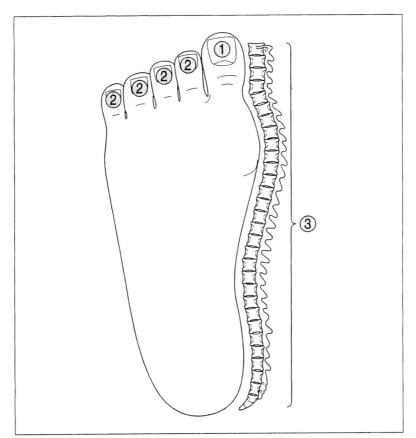

**FIGURE 6.17** *Pressure points on the top of the foot for treating overall balance. 1, brain reflex; 2, brain reflex; 3, spinal reflex.*

reflective point of the brain. The spinal column responds to the outer edge of the big toe to the instep down to the edge of the heel.

Pump the meridian on the top of the big toe 3 or 4 times. Then pump the tops of each toe separately, twice. You are working the reflex point for the brain that is on each toe. Gentle but firm pressure should be used.

Next you need to work the reflex points for the spinal column. They run along the outer edge of the big toe, down along the base and down the inner edge of the foot to the base of the heel. These are the meridian points for the entire spinal column. Move your thumb along the meridians by sliding down the outer edge of the client's big toe, continuing down the inside edge to the heel, very slowly. Then use tiny circles to work in an upward direction. Repeat the sliding down and circling back upward twice.

Repeat the entire process on the other foot. Ask if the client feels more at ease. If needed, repeat the entire process on both feet, 2 or 3 times. Give the client's body at least 10 to 12 minutes to respond. Remember that reflexology is effective, but it does take time to get the relay to the brain and back again.

### Client Profile

All clients can benefit from this session. This is particularly good to use on couples. I have found it easy to convince engaged couples to come in for sessions 2 weeks before their wedding. The tensions build so high that the overall balance treatment is perfect. Other excellent candidates are pregnant women, college students before examinations, and sales executives who are under pressure for heavy sales quotas. Get them to come in for a treatment at least once a week for the first 2 to 3 weeks. It is a judgment call, based on how severe their life stress is and for how long it has existed.

# Depression

If clients have serious or long-standing problems with depression, they need to seek medical assistance. No reflexologist should attempt to play "therapist." The reasons for a person to feel depressed can be as complex as we are unique individuals. Just handling the daily events of our lives will occasionally make us feel negative. We cannot expect every day to be a joy and feel "all at peace with the world." Listening to a daily news broadcast can make us feel uneasy so it is not surprising that we can feel depressed several times a day.

Many factors can cause people to become depressed. People try to assume their entire family's problems. They believe it is their job to solve everyone's dilemmas. These people are setting themselves up for discord and stress. With the trend of more American families having only one parent as the head of household, that parent is forced to take on much more responsibility than originally planned when they first decided to become a family. Single parents are great candidates for stress reduction. If they do not find a way to vent the pressures of everyday problems, they will develop signs of depression. Left unhandled, they can become fully depressed and begin a negative spiral downturn, making it impossible to run their household efficiently.

Depression can also come from dealing with anger. Some people will hold in their anger to the point that it begins to eat at them from the inside. Besides developing ulcers and blazing headaches, the anger causes the brain to shut down and depression begins.

These situations require professional assistance. Reflexologists can help reduce certain stress levels and offer a tranquil place to let clients truly relax. However, reflexologists must be aware that they will not be "solving the client's problems" through reflexology. They will be part of the much larger treatment the major element of the client's problem is out of the realm of reflexology. However, reflexology can assist in lessening depressed sensations. A trained reflexologist can offer a wonderful session that will bring about a feeling of ease and relaxation so that the client will leave feeling calmed. The severity of the reasons the client is depressed will determine how often sessions should be scheduled.

The reflexologist must be reasonably sure that the depression the client is complaining about is not a major problem such as manic/depressive tendencies caused by a brain chemical imbalance (that condition requires a drug prescription). Once it is established that the client does not have a serious medical problem and is just feeling a little low, the session can be started.

Begin with soft music and lower the lights. The atmosphere will help calm the client. Make sure that you change your voice to a very soft-spoken tone. By slowing down your speech, you will automatically create a more peaceful speaking voice. Most people will speed up their speech when they are edgy, out of sorts, or feeling pressure.

The reflexology session will concentrate on the nervous system. The key glands are the adrenal, pituitary, and the **pineal**. The diaphragm helps regulate a steadier breathing pattern and the voice. The brain is the main "boss" and needs some special TLC; because you cannot offer it any other way, reflexology is the best way to make it feel "at peace." You will work on all the meridian points for each of thcsc glands, the diaphragm, and the brain. It is advisable to work the ears, hands, and feet when treating the client for depression. If you want to work only one area, then do the feet.

### On the Ear

The main reflex point is for the brain, which is at the top of outer ridge of the ear. Work both ears at the same time. Place your thumb pad on the inside of the meridian point. Back the thumb with the support of your index finger by

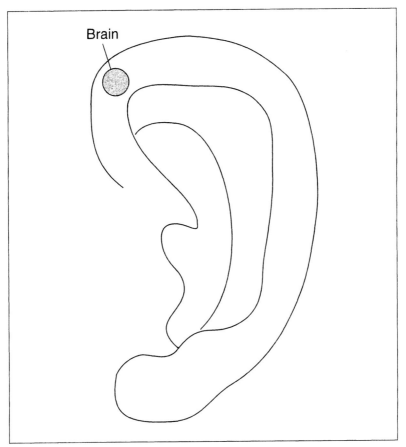

*FIGURE 6.18* *Pressure point on the ear for treating depression.*

placing it behind the ear. Hold the reflex point to the count of 5 and release.

### On the Hand

The reflex points you need to work on will be for the pituitary, pineal, and adrenal glands, the diaphragm, and the brain. Both hands will be manipulated. The meridian

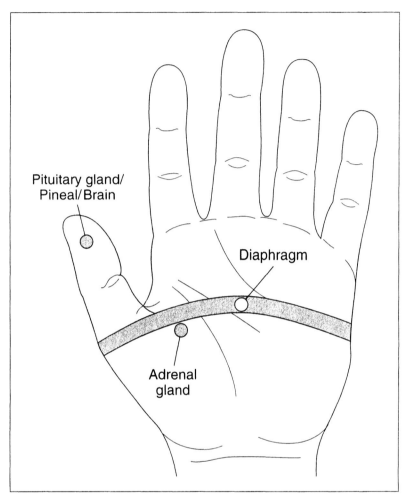

**FIGURE 6.19** *Pressure points on the palm for treating depression.*

point for the brain is at the top part of the thumb pad. The meridian for the pituitary and pineal glands is the same point, and it is in the center of the pad area. The diaphragm's meridian runs across the entire palm on both hands. The reflex point for adrenal glands is at the top part of the fleshy area beneath the base of the thumb on both hands. Checking with the diagram will aid you in finding these meridians.

Start the treatment session by working on the client's nondominant hand. You will work on both hands by the end of the session. Begin with the reflex for the brain. Place your thumb over it and apply a firm pumping action for 3 or 4 seconds. Then slide down to the meridian point for the pituitary and pineal glands. Pump this point with your thumb for 4 seconds. Then make 5 counter-clockwise circles over this point. Pump again for 3 seconds. Then reverse the movement to clockwise.

Slide your thumb down to the reflex for the adrenal gland, pump this one for 3 seconds, followed by 5 counter-clockwise circles. Pump again for 3 seconds, and reverse the movement to clockwise.

Lastly, slide your thumb to the center of the palm, and pump the meridian ribbon in the center point for 2 to 3 seconds. Then slide your thumb over the entire meridian ribbon from the inner edge to the outer 5 or 6 times, making small clockwise circles while you work from side to side.

## On the Foot

You will work on both feet, but start on the client's nondominant side. The brain reflex point is on the top of the big toe, on both feet. Pump this meridian 3 times and then over the top of every toe.

Slide down a short distance to the center of the fleshy part of the big toe, which is where the meridian point for the pituitary and pineal glands lies. Pump this point 4 times.

The diaphragm is at the very top of the arch, or for flat-footed people, it is at the bottom of the ball of the foot. Glide your thumb to the area at the top of the arch. This is where the diaphragm meridian ribbon lies. It is not a singular point. It flows from one side of the foot to the other. Place your thumb in its center point and pump it for 3 seconds. Then

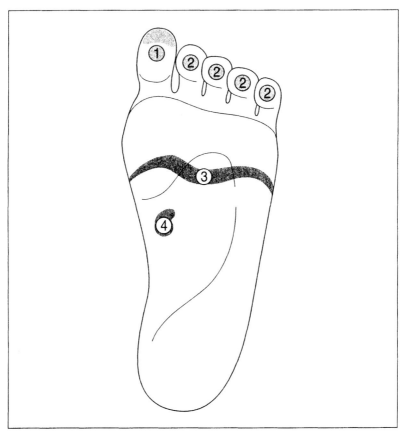

*FIGURE 6.20* Pressure points on the foot for treating depression. 1, pituitary/pineal/brain; 2, brain; 3, diaphragm; 4, adrenal gland.

work across the entire meridian ribbon by moving in counter-clockwise circles in one direction, and clockwise circles in the other.

The adrenal gland's meridian point is close to the diaphragm. Dividing the width of the foot in half, on the right foot it is slightly to the right of center; on the left foot it is close to the center. The diagram will help you find these meridians. Once you have located the meridian, pump it with your thumb with firm pressure for 5 or 6 seconds.

## Client Profiles

An example worth sharing comes through one of my personal clients. She had come in for reflexology sessions for overall balancing once a month for 6 years. Now she was going through court proceedings to gain a divorce and custody of her 3 children. During the week before the trial and through the 2 days of the court hearings, she came in every day for 1-hour sessions.

It was her opinion that the sessions were so helpful that she stayed composed throughout the court proceedings. She said that she would have otherwise broken down and cried throughout the entire process. She told me that the attorney and judge commented on her behavior and that it went favorably for her because she was able to show such a positive, well-defined role. The judge watched her ex-husband yell and tender some very negative comments at her. She remained cool, calm, and collected, never expressing any anger. She did not walk around depressed. Her children were calmer and less affected by what was going on because she was able to smile and laugh with them. She felt that she was able to keep her home a more normal and happy place because she was not dealing with depression. She said she would be forever thankful for having a way to get her body to release the tension and hostility that was inside.

Harriet came into the spa for a complete **body glow** and massage. She was unhappy about her children leaving home. Although she understood why they had to go, one for college and one for a great job opportunity, their departure made her depressed. While she was getting the sea salt rub, she mentioned it to her technician. This employee passed on the information to the massage therapist. When Harriet had her massage session, it was decided that she should have a reflexology treatment. Harriet was excited to learn that reflexology could help her feel less depressed, as long as she was willing to come in for a series of sessions. She was eager to do so.

## Constipation

Nearly everyone has had the sensation of not being able to move the bowels, called **constipation**. Some of the more common causes are:

- Various eating habits, such as eating very late at night
- Poor eating habits, including insufficient roughage or fiber in the diet
- Eating too quickly so that food is only partly chewed
- Life-style factors such as a high-stress job

Occasional **irregularity** is not usually a problem. The body's internal system will work it all out. However, for the person with a constant or daily bout of constipation, the problem exists. First, you should recommend that the client see an **internist** to ensure that a serious medical problem such as a blocked intestine, twisted colon, or early stages of colitis is not the cause of the constipation.

Constipation may be a side effect of many medications. Only a doctor can decide if the need for drugs outweighs the side effects the client may experience. Illness can also cause constipation, forcing bacteria counts to grow too high. This is another reason it is imperative that the client seeks medical attention if the constipation is not just a short-term, nonregular condition.

The reflexologist needs to ask a series of questions to have a better understanding of what the usual pattern of elimination was before the constipation started. The following are the most relevant ones.

1. When was the last time you had a complete bowel movement? Their answer should be sometime with the last 72 hours. If it has been more than 7 days, the client should see a doctor very quickly. The toxicity within the body will be extremely high and other infections can be brewing.

2. Do you have a regular time that your body wants to eliminate its solid wastes? Ideally, the client should be able to tell you a specific part of the day that the digestive system collects and removes the fecal material, such as when he or she wakes up, right before bedtime, or at a specific time of day, like 10:00 PM. If the client has had a fairly regular pattern, and only recently the pattern has changed, then the reflexologist will know that a pattern was present and something recent has caused it to change.

3. What is the client's diet? Does the client make the time to sit down and eat or are meals eaten on the run? Although you are not a nutritionist, you can have a solid background in the basics. Remember, the *Nutritionists' Almanac*[1] is a great reference guide.

Through the use of reflexology, the client can have relief of constipation in less than an hour. Usually the reaction to the session is under 30 minutes, but it may not be the total release of the bowel. There will be a flatulent reaction at first. The gas moves around the intestines and colon during the process of getting the feces out. The reflexology session triggers the release of the feces to move toward the anus. It will also relax the anus to allow the final removal of the feces.

---

[1]*Nutritionists' Almanac* (1995). New York: McGraw-Hill.

One of the best reasons to use reflexology is that it has no side effects as do all laxatives. Even the popular, widely advertised fiber grain additives have problems. They create a weakness in the intestinal walls and ascending colon, causing the individual to use the products daily just to be able to go to the bathroom at all. The goal is to get the client's system to function by itself. Reflexology allows the body a natural way to readjust itself and get back on track. The reflexologist has to work all the reflexes for the four parts of the colon—the ascending colon, the transverse colon, the descending colon, and the sigmoid colon—along with the large and small intestines, the ileocecal valve, and the anus.

The small intestine is made up of three parts:

1. The **duodenum** is where the contents of the stomach go to move toward the final elimination process. It is the top part of the small intestine.
2. The **jejunum** is where the heavy part of the digestion of the food material occurs. It is the middle section of the small intestine.
3. The **ileum** is where the small intestine connects with the large intestine. It is the lowest portion of the small intestine.

Between the large and small intestines is the connection called the **ileocecal valve**. Its main function is to keep the bacteria caught in the body's waste from going back up into the system. The large intestine separates the digested food into various waste materials. The fluids are sent to the bladder; the solid wastes are moved on through the system for final elimination.

### On the Hand
The hands and feet are the areas to work on. The feet are the first choice because the meridians on the feet are

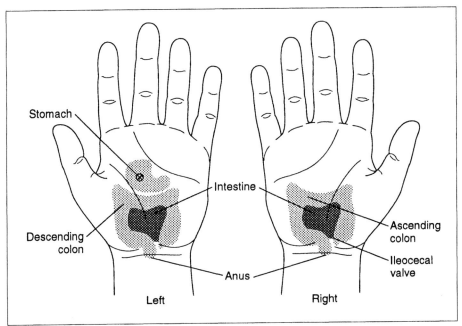

**FIGURE 6.21** *Pressure points on the hands for treating constipation.*

more reactive than those on the hands. On the hands the meridians are located as follows: the descending colon is on the left, next to the meridian for the intestines. The meridian for the descending colon is close to the inner edge of the palm, underneath the thumb. The large and small intestines are under the stomach reflex. They encompass the lower third of the palm area. The anus is at the bottom edge of the palm, right before the wrist area. It is the same on both hands. The meridian for the ascending colon is on the right hand on the outer edge of the palm, underneath the pinky finger. The reflex for the intestines is in the middle of the lower one-third of the palm area. But the ileocecal valve is on the right hand only. It has a singular meridian point that is located on the outer edge of the hand. Check the diagram for the exact location.

I advise you to begin work with the nondominant hand first. But because the reflex areas are found on both, you can begin on either hand. You should notice that there is not just a singular point, but rather a large area for the intestines and colon sections. Find the areas, as described above.

Start with the ascending colon reflex. Place your thumb pad over it as much as possible. Press very firmly, and hold the pressure to the count of 10. Release and then begin tiny clockwise circles over the area. Continue working the circles for 3 to 4 seconds. Then slide down to the intestinal reflex area. Apply firm pressure over it for 10 seconds. Release, and then begin tiny clockwise circles over the area. Continue working the circles for 3 seconds.

Slide over to the descending colon. Apply firm pressure over it for 10 seconds. Release and then begin tiny clockwise circles over the area. Continue working the circles for 3 seconds. Locate the anus meridian as described above. Place your thumb pad on it and pump the point for 5 to 7 seconds.

If you are working on the right hand, then locate the reflex for the ileocecal valve. Place your thumb pad on the reflex and pump the point to the count of 4. Stop and place constant pressure on the reflex for 3 seconds. Repeat this two-step process twice. Switch to begin working on the other hand. If you had been working on the left hand before, then do the ileocecal meridian now.

Next work with the reflective area for the intestines, as described above. Apply firm pressure over it for 10 seconds. Release, and then begin tiny clockwise circles over the area. Continue working the circles for 3 seconds. Slide over to the decending colon reflective area. Place your thumb pad over it as much as possible. Press very firmly, and hold the pressure to the count of 10. Release, and then begin tiny clockwise circles over the area. Continue working the circles for 3 to 4 seconds.

It should take about half an hour to take effect. Have your client relax and stay near a bathroom. The first reaction that the client will experience is the gas that has accumulated in the intestinal tract and colon. The fecal material will continue to process the gas even though it won't release out of the body. Clients occasionally release the gas during the treatment and become embarrassed. It is very important to make them understand that this is what their bodies need to do.

I have made it a policy to have an oscillation fan turned on before beginning the session. The air will move throughout the session and will minimize the discomfort of the client. Flatulence may not occur this quickly, but it will occur before the release is complete. Let clients know what is to happen so that they can be properly prepared.

### On the Foot

The feet are the stronger resource to get the release to occur. The same number of meridian points are engaged. Like the hands, you work both feet to do this treatment.

Because the right foot has the ileocecal valve meridian point, it would be good to start with the right foot. Begin with the transverse colon reflex located in the center of the arch. It is not a singular point, so place your thumb over the area and press firmly for 3 seconds. Release the pressure and switch to a pumping movement for the count of 3. Slide over to the meridian point for the ascending colon. Do the exact same movements you just completed on the transverse colon reflex.

The small intestine meridian area is right next to the ascending colon, but slightly over to the right. Place your thumb over the area and pump it for 5 to 6 seconds. Then move to the singular meridian point for the ileocecal valve. Apply firm pressure with your thumb pad on the point. Hold to the count of 6. Move down to the meridian point for the

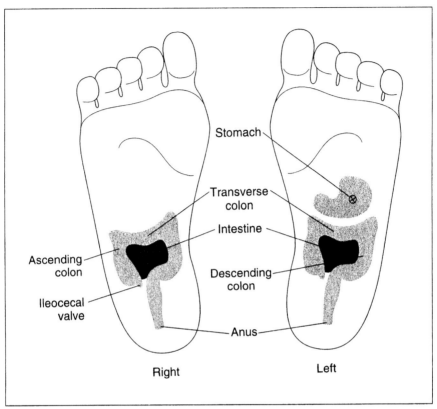

*FIGURE 6.22* Pressure points on the feet for treating constipation.

anus, located at the center of the base of the heel. Apply firm pressure to the count of 3. Release the pressure and make small clockwise movements directly on the point. Repeat the firm pressure and circles twice.

Now switch to the left foot. Begin with the transverse colon reflex point, located in the center of the arch. It is not a singular point, so place your thumb over the area and press firmly for 3 seconds. Release the pressure and switch to a pumping movement for the count of 3.

Slide over to the meridian point for the small intestine meridian area, which is right next to the descending colon, but slightly over to the left. Check the diagram for clarification of its exact location. Place your thumb over the area and pump it for 5 to 6 seconds. Still using your thumb pad, make small clockwise circles over the entire section. Move your thumb downward to the meridian for the anus, located at the center of the base of the heel. Apply firm pressure to the count of 3. Release the pressure and make small clockwise movements directly on the point. Repeat the firm pressure and circles twice.

### Client Profile

This is one of the most popular treatments. The reason is quite clear—the results are quick, and the relief priceless. OTC products are messy and often uncomfortable to use. Staying on high-fiber supplement is difficult on the internal organs and creates a dependency on bulk additives. They also increase the flatulence problem that often accompanies constipation.

Once it is determined that the constipation is not caused by a serious medical condition, the reflexology sessions are started. Each client will need a different program. There are no set patterns of treatment as can be used for other conditions. Let the client's body be the judge for the frequency of the sessions.

This treatment is appreciated by men as well as women, although most men will not admit to having a problem. This treatment should be done in private rather than in view of the other clients and coworkers, mainly because of the passing of gas from the intestines during the session. The more privacy you can offer, the better chance you will have getting the client to return. Flatulence may be a natural biologic event, but it embarrasses nearly everyone.

## *Summary*

This chapter is the most difficult in the book. No matter from which area of professional training you approach reflexology, the information in this chapter is what makes your business successful. None of you can expect to read this chapter once and understand all of it. The material will have to be read and studied. You will need to keep this chapter at your side as a guide for the first year of your work as a reflexologist. It would be a good idea to copy the pages and cover each page in plastic so that the print does not get hard to read after a while. You may work with oils and they will get into the fibers of the paper and make reading the material more difficult. Because the actual treatment sessions are what will make you a success in the field of reflexology, study this chapter well.

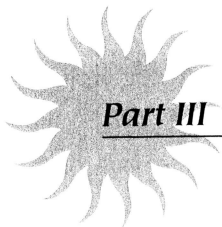

# Part III

# THE BUSINESS
# OF REFLEXOLOGY

# *Chapter Seven*

# BUSINESS
# CONSIDERATIONS

## *Overview*

This chapter provides you the specific details for creating a successful reflexology business. You need to know how to develop an exciting program of treatments that will keep the customers coming back for many of your fine services over a long period of time. The many different parts of operating a successful reflexology service business are fully explained. You will have to study this chapter carefully to grasp all its content. However, the time and effort will make your business more successful.

## *Introduction*

The reflexologist must be able to determine a plan for conducting services. As in any business, there are more elements to being successful than just learning the specific trade. The reflexologist must learn how to keep the clients coming back for many sessions. The old accounting rule applies: "Eighty percent of the business comes from 20% of the clients." In the reflexology business, this means that repeat visits are essential.

### How Do You Begin a Treatment?

It would not be a professional approach to have customers walk into the salon, place them in a chair or lounge, and jump into the treatment. You must make your clients feel special. For you to be successful, your clients must develop a sense of trust about your interest in them. Establishing a rapport with clients is vital to completing a successful treatment. The quicker that you can establish a relationship based on trust and warm communication, the faster you will create a client forever.

Every treatment session should begin with a firm handshake and a warm genuine smile. This may be the client's first session, or the individual may have seen other reflexologists before meeting you. Your treatment technique can be as individual as your own uniqueness. Listening to the client's reactions to any other sessions will aid you in creating a great treatment experience for that client. Remember, you want this client to want to return for many other sessions. One of the reasons should be because you paid attention to the client's specific needs. You were able to make this person feel special, an opportunity not often available in our normal routines.

When clients come to you for reflexology sessions, you have the unique opportunity to let them leave your salon feeling great and sensing that you care about them and their health. These may sound like simple words, but to clients who receive these messages, their entire outlook for the rest of the day may be changed. It is a powerful tool and as a reflexologist, you should use it as much as possible.

Not everything done during a reflexology session will be loving and gentle. It is important to keep in mind that parts of the reflexology session may be uncomfortable for the client. Some of the meridian points may be very tender to the touch. Most often you will find that an overworked meridian point and connecting nerve pathways register pain when pressed. This is a common occurrence and you want your client to accept it. You want your client to relax and understand that the momentary negative reaction will have a possible side effect—bringing about a more balanced body. The cliché "No pain, no gain" mildly fits this situation. Just because the meridian points may be tender, do not get callous about the real discomfort the client feels. Remember that everyone has a different tolerance for mild discomfort and you must work within the range of each client's tolerance level. To do otherwise is the fastest way to lose your business. When first establishing yourself in an area, keep in mind that everyone you come in contact with will know at least five other people they can tell about your work. It is totally up to you if they report a positive or negative experience!

You decide if you are to work on the client's ear, hand, or foot. In one session, it is not advisable to do all three areas on the first-time client. Because the foot has the most reflective meridian points, it is wise to begin all new clients there. Depending on the amount of time allotted for the client's session, it may not be appropriate to work on all three areas on repeat clients either.

### First-Time Clients

For a first-time client, you should gauge your time as follows: three-quarters of the session devoted to the exploratory phase and one-quarter to the implementation phase. Understanding the client's life-style and meridian points leads to a good treatment. Rushing through the process will only cause you to offer poor assistance in balancing the client's body. In addition, the exploratory is not painful, and the client's trust in you rises.

## What Record Keeping Is Needed for Each Client?

Whether you have only a single session or arrange for a series of treatment sessions, you must have accurate files on every client. The records should contain general information about the client. Specific information about the client will come during the exploratory phase of the session.

## Client History Form

Before you begin your session, have the client complete a client history sheet. A sample form follows, with explanations and clarifications for the reflexologist at the end of the form.

---

### Client History

1. Date: _____

2. Name: _____

3. Address: _____

4. City: _____ Zip: _____

5. Phone number: (      ) _____

6. Where did you hear about our
   services? _____

7. Do/Have any of your friends or relatives come to
   us for a session? _____

8. Is this your first reflexology session? _____

9. If not, when was your last one done? _____

10. By whom? _____

11. What was your reaction to the
    treatment? _____

12. Was there one particular part that was your
    favorite? _____

13. Was there a part of the session that was your
    least favorite? _____

14. What specifically brought you in to see us
    today? _____

---

15. Are you taking any medicines? If yes, what is the name of the medication and why was it prescribed? _____
Is it a long-term prescription or just for a few days? _____

16. Are you undergoing any chemotherapy? _____

17. Are you undergoing any radiation treatment? _____

18. Are you epileptic? _____ If yes, is your medicine regulated, or are you still working with your doctor to get it balanced? _____

19. Are there any other medical conditions that we should be made aware of at this time? _____
(e.g., having any metal plates or shunts in your body)

20. (optional) Please provide us with your doctor's name and phone number: _____

21. Do you smoke? _____ How much? _____

22. How regular are your sleeping habits? _____

23. How many hours do you sleep each night? _____

24. Do you get enough sleep nightly? _____

25. If not, why do you think you are not sleeping well?
_____

26. How much water do you drink per day? _____

27. How much caffeine do you consume? _____

28. Do you drink socially? _____

29. Do you eat a balanced diet? _____

General comments concerning questions on the Client's History form:

- Because reflexologists are not nutritionists, they should be careful not to present themselves as such. General healthy guidelines are easy to offer. You should make yourself knowledgeable about healthy life-style eating habits. Make sure that your clients are not left with the opinion that you are suggesting specific diet programs. It is advisable to gain as much knowledge on nutrition as possible. This author highly recommends *The Nutrition Almanac* (see page 119). This book is written in clear, simple terms and makes a lot of difficult information easy to understand. Keep this book with your *Physicians' Desk Reference* (*PDR*)[1]. Having it at fingertip access during a client's session provides you the ability to answer your client's questions about their diet without making false statements, or worse, giving bad advice that will jeopardize your client's health.

- Heavy drinking patterns need professional help. You cannot aid them except to suggest that the client look into assistance by a trained medical practitioner. The typical weekend drinker will show results of this pattern of alcohol consumption in the meridian points. You can localize them, but you cannot change the effects of alcohol toxicity. It is out of your range of treatment. Caffeine has a direct effect on the adrenal gland. It can also have a negative effect on the stomach lining.

- The guideline of eight 8-oz glasses of water consumed daily is not often followed. Juices can help fill in the shortage. Coffee, teas, and soft drinks all

---

[1]*Physicians' Desk Reference* (1996). Montvale, NJ: Medical Economics Company.

have water in them, but they also have other elements, such as caffeine, carbonation, and chemical ingredients that limit the ability of the water to truly hydrate the body. Pure water can make its way throughout every molecule of the body. Remember that intravenous feeding is sugar water being put directly into the veins. You would be helping your clients by making them understand the value of water consumption.[2]

- The standard is 8 hours of sleep, but not everyone needs the same amount. Many senior citizens sleep less than younger adults. Babies and growing children need more sleep. Keep an open mind and ask your clients to rate how well they feel they sleep. Four hours of solid sleep offers more than 8 hours of a restless sleep pattern.

- Many reports have shown that a consistent sleeping schedule creates a more regulated body function.

- The current trend in society is to be antismoking. I understand the better choice is to be a nonsmoker. However, I also know that it will not be popular to make a smoker feel ostracized by this opinion. Let your clients feel comfortable by being nonjudgmental

---

[2]A healthy water drinking schedule. I designed the following program in 1980 to help my skin care clients get used to drinking water daily:

For the first 2 days, drink one additional glass of water in addition to everything else you drink on a daily basis.
On the third day, drink two glasses. Do so for 2 more days.
On the fifth day, increase to three glasses for 3 consecutive days.
Then drink four glasses for 4 days.
Drink five glasses for 5 days. At this point, the client's tongue will create a thirsty feeling, thus making it easy to remember to drink the water.
Drink six glasses for 6 days.
Drink seven glasses for 7 days.
Finally, drink eight glasses for 8 days.

This program takes 6 weeks. The client will appreciate the results and not find it difficult to keep it up.

Using a beautiful crystal glass will make the whole process more enjoyable. The cut glass will attract the client, thus making it a subtle reminder to pick it up and take a drink.

about their life-style choices. This will allow them to be comfortable in disclosing other possibly difficult information about their health status. Your clients must be made to feel that you are not being judgmental about their lives.

• By having medical information on file, you will have a better understanding of the clients' internal care and the opportunity to establish a working relationship with a doctor for the future.

• I highly recommend having a copy of the *Physicians' Desk Reference* at your work station. The client will be impressed that you are professional enough to look up all medications.

## What Record Keeping Is Needed During Each Session?

The above questions and any others that you want to ask should be recorded on a file card. Although it is not necessary for the actual reflexology session, taking notes on the private information about the client can be done on the same record file. I am not known for my exceptional memory and, in fact, I have a terrible time remembering fine details. To compensate for this shortcoming, I record information about my client so that I can reread it before the client arrives. I record personal information such as:

• Client's birthday
• Anniversary date; how many years married
• How many children; their names and ages
• Where they have gone on any recent vacations
• Are they planning a family trip soon, and where are they going?

These questions are not too personal, but they give you something to talk about to the client that shows interest in the client's activities. Clients are often impressed that you remember these details. Obviously, do not make it known that you were reading your notes. Let it appear that the details just flow out of your head.

I also recommend that you send out birthday and anniversary cards a week before the date. This will give clients reason to think of you too and then make an appointment for a treatment. For the husbands of your clients, send a note before their anniversary date to suggest a special present for their wives. Getting a suggestion for a service from you as a "gift of love" will make them very happy. The wives love it too.

A 5 x 7 file card will do nicely. Taking notes in an abbreviated form will provide you with more space to keep your files orderly and manageable. You will be updating each client's file on every visit. I have found another benefit to keeping notetaking short—it prevents others from having access to personal information. Salons are not medical offices. The staff may not keep their gossip chatter out of the salon. You would not want your client to be able to read another client's card either. I have adopted a system that provides a form of cryptic notes that make perfect sense to me, and me alone.[3]

---

[3]Cryptic Note System. You are free to adapt any part of this system for all client record note taking. This works for hairdressers, estheticians, masseuses, and reflexologists. Here is an example: S, NS, SCD=0, G=4, CF=3, No Med, No Allg, Sleep/ +, 6. This reads: Single, Non-smoker, a zero Social Casual Drinker, consumes four glasses of water, three cups of coffee, takes no medications, and has no known allergies, sleeps well for six hours.

S = single; D = divorced; D w/# = divorced with a number of children still living with them; S/Nic = a regular smoker consuming nicotine; NS = nonsmoker; SCD = social casual drinking; G = amounts of water consumed; CF = coffee; No Med = no medications; No Allg = no known allergies; Sleep/+ = good sleeping pattern; Sleep/- = poor sleeping patterns or tough getting a regular sleeping habit; L-h/TT = left-handed and very tender to touch, needs a gentle approach; R-h/RT = right-handed and does not need a gentle approach; +Att = client has a positive mental attitude; -Att = client has a negative mental attitude.

Then I use a smile symbol to represent whether I enjoy them or a frown to indicate a "challenging" client that takes more of my energy.

## *Summary*

The sign of really successful reflexologists is how busy their business' are on a regular basis. Keeping excellent records on your clients will allow you to track the peaks and valleys of your scheduling. It also gives you information to plan for the future growth of your practice.

You need to know the best times to plan your own time-off, such as a vacation. Keeping records on each client lets you know when they are most likely to come see you. Obviously, you do not want to be leaving on a trip when your most loyal clients will be wanting to have some work done.

Reflexologists have to make themselves stick to accurate record keeping and client retention records so that they will be able to see the "bottom line" grow each and every year.

# Chapter Eight

## MARKETING IDEAS FOR THE PROFESSIONAL

## Overview

All successful professionals must have a business plan to keep their doors open. Many beauty professionals are very talented, but lack the accounting and retailing skills to make their talents grow into a viable business. This chapter offers specific suggestions on how to plan for your future. It gives you the individual programs that were used for many years in my thriving practice. All the information has been tested and proven to be effective. Besides bringing you more than 17 years of expertise in reflexology, I have a Bachelor's degree in accounting and Master's degrees in marketing and management. You are provided key facts and information available only through these college degree programs.

## Introduction

Through years of business accounting evaluations, the following statistic has been proven to be accurate for every single service-directed business. All hairdressing, esthetics, manicuring, and massage businesses are service directed. Eighty percent of your business comes from 20% of your clientele. The larger the clientele base you can create the more substantial your financial earning power will be. When I lecture worldwide, I use the phrase "Work smarter, not harder."

Using this accounting principal, you can develop a client base that will keep your budgets from peaking and then plummeting. Most of us who work in the beauty industry work on commission. Because this allows us the opportunity to share in all of our hard work, we usually love the arrangement. It can be difficult to live comfortably on a budget when the revenues coming in are not the same all of the time.

## Marketing Strategies

All across the country, the effects of the seasons will create influxes of traffic patterns that will either benefit or hinder our financial status. Certain holidays like Christmas or Easter bring people into our salon. Summer vacations and the dead of winter keep clients preoccupied in other directions. In areas like Florida, they have a unique condition called the "Snow Bird Months." During this time, the residents from cold climate states will come to Florida to live during the harsh winter season. The population of Southern Florida can double, based on the severity of the winter storms. In the beauty business, this can mean feast or famine for clientele activity.

Effective marketing will be the key to your success. Here are some of the marketing programs that I have used to create my business. In 17 years, the programs have been tried, revised, and reinstituted. The results of each are also being offered. Please take this information and adapt any or all for your own use.

## Gift Certificates

Although the idea is not original, every major salon carries some sort of gift certificate program. It is typical to see signs set out in the salon, usually at the receptionist desk, saying "Gift Certificates Are Available." During the Christmas holiday season, most salons put a stronger emphasis on them for obvious reasons.

I have created specific gift certificates that are printed in advance. Then with a gold or silver calligraphy pen, I personalize them for the client. In addition, I have small note cards made up in script style printing; I can easily add the client's name to the card, expressing my interest in seeing that person for the specific treatment. The card has a brief description of why the service would fill the client's needs. Remember, benefits do not sell the product as much as the "wants" of the client.

The following layout of a typical benefits statement versus a wants statement might help you to see the difference. For this example you have a gift certificate for a half-hour reflexology hand treatment.

---

This reflexology hand treatment will allow exploration of all the meridian points in your hands. Your reflexologist will be able to rebalance the meridian reflexes with an effective pressure point massage. Working your meridian reflexes will set into motion a wonderful chain reaction in your circulatory system.

(Key benefits: rebalancing the reflex points and reaction in the circulatory system)

---

This reflexology hand treatment will relax you by having your reflex points gently manipulated. You will feel calmer and in good spirits when the session is completed.

(Key wants: to be relaxed, calm, and in good spirits)

---

This does not tell as much about what reflexology is, but it lets the client know the positive effects of receiving a treatment.

When new clients come into the salon for any service, you should ask them for their birthday, month and day only.

Then send them a birthday gift certificate. It can be as simple as a 5- to 10-minute reflexology exploratory. The idea that you are sending them a gift on their birthday is important, whether or not it is for a service that they would normally use. In fact, offering them an opportunity to try something new in the salon is a better marketing strategy than giving them a gift certificate for something they already use.

I do not believe in giving away services just to get a new customer to walk in the door. An effective slant on the give-away is to offer the "buddy system." Two people can come in together to get the same treatment. They share in the experience, and they split the price. In effect, you are discounting your service price by 50%. But unlike offering anyone half-off for a service, you get the opportunity to meet and work with two people at the same time (not the exact same moment, just close together). This makes for easier bonding with both people. They get to chat about you and your business to all of their friends. And they get to share a pleasant few hours or day together. Women love to chat about new events and experiences; having one to share and talk about to others makes for an irresistible combination.

## Personal Shopper

Men have a difficult time shopping for the women in their lives. If you can fill their shopping needs, you will have a loyal customer. I created the "Professional Shopper Service" just for my male clientele. My male clients list all of their family relatives and the reasons that they need to purchase them presents. All birthdays, anniversaries, holidays, and any other occasions, such as graduations, weddings, newborn arrivals are listed. Then they provide the specific dates of each occasion. In addition, a few key questions are asked about each person they need to make a purchase for.

- Does the man consider the woman to be conservative or moderate in the way she dresses?

- Is the woman likely to read a romance novel or a murder mystery?
- Does the person prefer the smell of roses or the smell of the ocean?

The answers guide me in selecting the gifts.

Next, I ask for a budget allowance and make sure that the man feels in total control of the money to be spent. It is important that they not feel that you expect a certain amount of money to be used. Any amount of money can work. It is vitally important to stay within the allotted amount; never go over unless you are willing to absorb the difference yourself! The beauty of the system is that it makes the man feel that he is selecting the "best money can buy." He is not having to do the shopping himself and he gets all the accolades from the recipient.

All of the gift certificates are for services, but included will always be some kind of product—something they can see, hold, and touch. A strong effort is made to choose products normally sold in the salon. However, if an item that would be perfect for the client is not available in the salon, I go out and purchase it. The man covers all costs. Everything is beautifully gift wrapped. The man is given the option of selecting his own personal card or I make one on the computer. You could make an arrangement with an independent card broker to get unique and different kinds of cards if you do not have access to the desk-top capabilities of a computer.

Except for the major holidays I personally deliver the gifts to the man's office. At busy times like Christmas, the gifts are prepared and held in the salon for the men to pick up. The salon looks more festive and the gifts plant the idea of the gift certificates and presents in the minds of other customers. Even people walking by can notice the lovely packages and come in to inquire about the "Personal Shopping Service."

### "Please Forgive Me" Gift Certificates

Reflexology is a terrific way to say "I'm sorry." Because of the immediate sense of well-being and pleasant neural response to the treatment, reflexology can make people feel positive when they leave the business location, even if they arrived feeling glum and negative. The gift certificates I created are in three forms.

**The "I Wish We Could Make Up" Certificate.** This is for those who had a minor tiff with someone they care about. This is a 15-minute treatment, where half the time is spent on the exploratory and the other on a mild implementation phase.

**The "Boy Did I Mess Up" Certificate.** This is designed for people who made a mistake and cannot change it but feel badly about doing it and would like to get back into the good graces of another person. This works for personal relationships and business associates too. This is a 30-minute session, in which besides the more thorough exploratory there is a concentration on the endocrine system during the implementation phase to release the endorphins to make the recipient feel calmer and less negative.

**The "Will You Ever Forgive Me?" Certificate.** For those in trouble with their significant other, this is the perfect gift to make them want to "kiss and make up" afterward. This is a full-hour session, in which attention is given to the overall balance treatment along with working all meridians responding to the endocrine system. I recommend that the purchaser plan this appointment for his or her mate. Then the purchaser is advised to make plans to follow the session with a romantic dinner—and the rest is up to them.

## Added Value

If you sell body beauty products in your business, adding gift certificates for any of the reflexology treatments will increase your sales. This is particularly helpful if retail locations around your business sell bath and body products at a fraction of what you charge. With the reflexology gift certificate added to the value, the customer's interest in selecting your products will increase.

I do not believe in giving services away for free. The idea that customers will pay for something after it was given to them for nothing just has not proven to be true. Giving away "freebies" gets people in the door, but the policy does not create long-term clients. What does work for me is offering additional value for no additional out-of-pocket costs. I prefer to give customers a retail product at no charge if they book a service. The retail product never cost me much money. The customers have another reason to return, once they have used all the product. Customers get more for their money, but still pay for the service.

There is one situation that does make giving a reflexology service away for free valuable for client retention. On existing good customers, ones who are coming in steadily for other services, it works to offer a complimentary treatment. They already know and like your business. They will be coming back no matter what service is given away. Introducing them to a new service, free of charge, will give you the opportunity to expand the services that they will book in the future. This also has an added benefit of giving them first-hand experience in a service that they might buy as a gift for someone else. When an introduction of a service is being offered, I always inquire if they know someone who might like this service as a gift.

Giving away services brings to mind the idea about giving away product samples. I do not agree with the notion that if you give away a prepackaged sample, the customer will come in when it is used up to purchase a full-sized one. It has been my experience that it does not work that way at all. To remedy this situation, I do the following. I take a full-sized container off the retail shelf and show it to the customers. This gives them eye contact with the product I want them to purchase. I go over the information on the label. Then I squeeze a small amount into a clean, unmarked plastic sample container, which can be purchased in bulk. I give customers enough product to use daily for 4 days. I promise to call them at the end of a week. This is enough time for them to have used it all. I will ask them their opinion of how it worked to let them know that I will be following their progress with the new product. It also lets them know that they will be hearing from me soon and makes them feel that they should indeed try the sample, rather than just placing in a drawer.

It is usually cheaper for me to take a retail product and place small amounts of the product in a plastic container than to buy the sample sizes from the manufacturer. With all the labeling requirements of sample packs, the manufacturer must pass on the high costs to you. By showing and discussing the product ahead of time with the customer you have informed them of the required information. Now they cannot take the sample to a competitor and get them to give them their version of your selected product. I know that this is a common practice because my clients bring me their samples and ask me what I have that is similar. I then sell them my selection!

## Advertising

Placing a good ad in your local Yellow Pages directory will be one of the best ways to spend your advertising dollars. When people are looking in the Yellow Pages, they are seeking some business or service. You have a willing participant for your customer files.

Not all Yellow Pages are the same in their direct benefits to the area. Call around your location and ask the owner of another kind of business which Yellow Pages they use. As long as they are in your locale, it is a safe bet that you would get satisfactory coverage using the same company.

Most often it is the local phone company's Yellow Pages that will give you the best results.

> **NOTE:** Take the time to create interesting written copy for your ad. Remember that people's wants drive them to make purchases, not product and service benefits. Create your ad around filling those wants.

Look at your local competition. What grabs your attention? It is probably a good guess that it will grab someone else's too. Use a professional writer and design artist if you can. If you are on a budget, seek out the assistance of all family and friends who can help put the ad together. Another excellent source is your local college. Contact their creative writing department and the art department director. Paying students to do the job allows them to use the work as proof of their skills, thus adding to their portfolio. You get the work done for much less than you could otherwise. If you have a large assignment, you can talk to the teacher of a specific class and ask if he or she would consider making your ad a class project. Not only will you get many more ideas, but everyone who knows the group of students will learn about your business. It is an indirect form of networking that is powerful.

## Expiration Dates

Another point in advertising and promotions is the expiration date for the offer. Always put a limit to how long a promotion or special will last. Put it in clear, visible writing on a sign at the front desk or on the mirror in the bathroom and dressing areas. A good rule of thumb is to keep the amount of time to come in for a service at 30 days or less. If the customer is not motivated to come in at first, waiting longer will not change the interest level.

Gift certificates should always have expiration dates. Thirty, 60, and 90 days are the usual. Some people let them go for 6 months. I feel that makes for poor tracking and lack of business revenue from future leads from the gift certificate. It also lessens the likelihood that the gift certificate will actually be used.

## Networking

The traditional forms of networking can be valuable. Attending the local chapter of the Chamber of Commerce gets you a certain amount of exposure. You might find a company that is willing to do **trades** with you. As a reflexologist who can reduce stress levels in their clients' lives, you will get interest from other business owners. Local chapters of the service clubs and other business groups all have regular meetings, usually breakfast or luncheon sessions. Most of them list their meetings in the calendar section of the local paper. Most groups will allow you to come in as a guest once before asking you to join.

For those of you who are female business owners, a local chapter of the American Business Women's Association is a terrific place to meet others like yourself. This group is especially receptive to joint events.

## Donations

Donations can get out of hand. If you are looking for an effective way to get donations to work for you, try any of the following.

Charities hold benefits to raise money. They will create a program or newsletter to publicize their event. If you are not aware which organizations are active in your local area, check with the editor of the local paper. You want to connect with an organization that does numerous newspaper announcements. This will add to your exposure. You will be able to cut out the newspaper clippings and have them in your business for your clients to see. It's not right to "blow your own horn," but they will get the message by seeing the connection between you and them.

For some of you, offering a cash donation is not going to be easy. But because you are a beauty professional, you have services that they will need to make the key organizers look good on the day of the special event. Hair styling, manicures, pedicures, facials, and makeup are all needed to look perfect. You have to arrange donating your time and expertise in exchange for getting your business advertised in their announcement. In a way it is a form of **bartering** that can work well for everyone.

Besides finding local charity organizations, there are other opportunities to gain recognition and public support. Local high schools or community colleges put on theater productions every year. Take an ad in their programs. Every student gets one, plus all of their friends and family learn of your business. They appreciate your support of the school production. Again, if cash expenditures are the problem, you can volunteer your time to teach the students how to do their makeup and hair for the production. If you volunteer to do the work for them, they usually give you recognition on the credits. If you have some older inventory that you are having trouble selling, donate it to the school's theater production group. (Another worthwhile way to get rid of older cosmetics or products is to donate them to a local nursing home.)

## Group Meetings

If you have any talent for public speaking, you can offer to lecture to any women's group meeting. These organizations are always looking for speakers and new topics. Having you lecture and demonstrate any part of the reflexology system will greatly benefit everyone. It will definitely develop a relationship between you and the audience. Reflexology is a topic that is easy to "show" and fun for audience participants. A large diagram of the feet and hands is all you need to make a lecture eye-catching and informative.[1]

## Joint Offerings

Marketing yourself with other businesses in your area is usually an effective way to gain popularity. It is important to choose a business that already has a wonderful reputation in the area. Take it from my personal experience, researching the company before you approach it is well worth the effort.

Here's what happened to me. I had opened a new holistic health skin care business in a city that I had not lived in for very long. Therefore, I did not know the "lay-of-the-land," so to speak. Nearby was a fitness business that appeared to be very busy. I called ahead to make an appointment with the manager to discuss doing some referral business together. I went in and on first impression, it looked wonderful. The place was brightly lit and clean and had many people walking around. I was greeted warmly, at first. When I said that I had a business appointment with the manager, the attention previously given to me ceased. I should have been aware of this obvious change and sent a message to my own brain.

The manager was pleased with my suggestions, which were as follows. I would provide the center with premade certificates for their members to come into my salon as a guest of the fitness business. It would be as though the center had "paid" for them to come in for a service. I thought that I could then have the opportunity to sell myself to the customer for future services. In addition, I would offer

---

[1]Several sources for the charts are listed in the back of this book. Digits International has one of the finest charts on the market. If you do not want to purchase one, you can copy one from a textbook in any library.

the fitness staff complimentary services to let them personally experience the services that I wanted their customers to use. I figured they could "talk up" my business if they had some first-hand knowledge about what I did.

At the outset it seemed like a win-win situation. Here's what went wrong. The manager used my "free employee" service certificates as a means to get employees to meet their sales quotas. Only those who reached the mark could get them, and those who did it consistently received more than one. This made for ill will with other employees. This I did not know until much later on, too much later.

The customers they had "hustled" to sign up felt that my business tactics would be similar and decided not to use the certificates at all. Probably the concept "Nothing is for nothing" crossed their minds. The fitness business had a reputation in the area as a hard-sell operation. Since I was new to the area, I did not have a clue to what the residents thought of them. The fitness firm probably did a lot of business with other new people like me. But once they were hustled, they were less likely to put themselves in that "pressure" situation again.

This promotion went on for 3 months. It took almost a full month to realize something was not working as I had expected. I was obligated to honor the certificates and they had a 90-day expiration. After that experience, it was refreshing to learn how to do it right. That knowledge came from the American Business Women's Association, which is particularly open to the idea.

## *Summary*

Very few handbooks will give you the technical information to do a specific service and offer the marketing support to make a complete package. The old adage "It's not always what you know that makes you a success" is clearly understood in this chapter. Learning how to implement your training is essential. However, learning how to get people to know that you are a specialist is just as important. In the first 3 years of your business, it may be even more valuable than the skill itself.

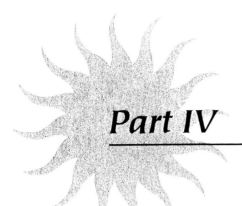

# Part IV

## APPENDICES

# *Appendix A*

# TERMS AND DEFINITIONS

**Acupressure point massages:** An ancient Chinese massage. A special form of massage that uses all the meridian points throughout the body to release negative synapses with the use of firm pressure. Most often performed with the finger pads and thumb.

**Adrenal gland:** One of a pair of ductless glands, located above the kidneys, consisting of a cortex and a medulla. A major contributor to the body's energy level.

**Anemia:** A condition in which the blood is deficient in red blood cells, in hemoglobin, or in total volume. The condition weakens the body's defenses against bacteria and viruses. This makes the person more susceptible to colds, flu, and other minor sicknesses. Iron supplements will increase the number of red blood cells.

**Bartering:** A method of obtaining products or services by swapping with another company or person their products or services. No money is used. It is part of the "trades" that companies set up.

**Body glow:** A term used in day spas to explain a method of removing dead skin cells from the entire body. A form of exfoliation is used by the technician on the client. Usually it is in a form of sea salt or herbal scrubs, such as almond meal and honey. It is rubbed over the client's skin and wiped off. Then a film of oil is applied over the skin to leave it silky smooth.

**Cancer:** A serious disease requiring immediate medical attention. It is the process in which the body produces more white blood cells than red blood cells, and they begin to attack the body from the inside. It produces tumors and lesions that quickly grow and consume healthy tissue within the body. Although some forms of cancer are less life-threatening than others, no cancerous cells should be ignored.

**Cellular rejuvenation:** The process of renewing the cells of the body. Most often refers to the skin cells within the stratum corneum layer of the epidermis.

**Cervical:** The top part of the spinal column. There are seven vertebrae in this portion. The first is the atlas, which holds up the skull. The second is the axis, which allows the head to turn to either side. The seventh vertebra is at the base of the neck.

**Coccyx:** Also referred to as the tail bone, it is the very end of the vertebral column. It terminates in the top section of the back of the pelvis region of the body.

**Constipation/irregularity:** The condition in which the person is not able to release the bowels/feces in a normal amount of time. The human body usually rids itself of fecal matter in regular periods of time, such as 24 to 72 hours. If the body does not empty the bowel in less than 3 days, the person is said to be constipated. If a normal pattern for waste removal is not systematic, the person is considered to be irregular.

**Descending colon:** One of the four parts of the colon tract, it is located on the left side of the abdomen. It handles the waste material after it has traveled through the ascending colon and moves the feces to the sigmoid colon.

**Diaphragm:** A muscular membranous partition separating the thoracic cavity from the abdominal cavity. It vibrates when receiving or producing sound waves.

**Diabetes:** A disease of the pancreas. The pancreas stops producing insulin, and the body is not able to break down sugar molecules. This disease requires medical attention! Side effects of the disease affect the patient in many different ways. Circulation of the blood is adversely affected. Extreme caution must be exercised when working on a client with diabetes. It is highly recommended that you receive permission from the assigned doctor before any treatment sessions are started.

**Duodenum:** The upper portion of the small intestine. The duodenum lies right next to the stomach and accepts the food for continuing the process of digestion.

**Duodenal ulcer:** A hole in the lining of the upper part of the small intestine caused by the highly powerful stomach acid dripping into the lining.

**Epidermis:** The top layer of the skin. One of three layers of the skin.

**Esophagus:** A muscular tube that leads from the pharynx to the stomach, passes down the neck between the trachea and spinal column. It is about 9 inches long.

**Esthetic hug:** A term I coined to describe a two-handed handshake that I use with every client. I use this handshake to show my interest in my clients and to make them comfortable with my coming into their personal space. It is a way of getting a nonverbal permission to work on them.

All of my services require physical contact of some kind. Facials, reflexology, waxing, or makeup all require body contact.

**Esthetician:** A licensed professional trained in skin care and makeup techniques. Usually performs various services within the beauty industry. Some of the more popular ones are facials, waxing (removal of unwanted hair by methods other than electrolysis), body contouring, glycolic acid peels, and reflexology.

**Fallopian tubes:** A pair of slender tubes leading from the body cavity to the uterus; they transport ova from the ovary to the uterus during the time when the female is able to conceive a child.

**Fetal position:** The position of the unborn baby while in the mother's womb. The exact curve of the spine, head, and buttocks while inside the womb.

**Flatulence:** Intestinal gas. To pass a lot of gas through the anus, creating strain on the internal organs, along with noticeable odor and sounds.

**Hangover:** A term used to describe the headache, nausea, stomach distress, and overall negative sensations after consuming too much alcohol. The alcohol gets into the bloodstream and poisons it, causing the body to revolt against the toxins created. It is particularly detrimental to the brain because the alcohol directly affects its functions.

**Happy hour:** The time a bar will offer special rate drinks to entice customers to frequent their establishment, usually immediately after working hours, 5:00 PM to 7:00 PM.

**Hemorrhoids:** A mass of dilated tortuous veins in swollen tissue situated at or within the anal area.

**Ileocecal valve:** Connection between small and large intestines.

**Ileum:** Lowest portion of small intestine, connects to large intestine.

**Infomercials:** These are half-hour TV commercials that sell a product or service to the public. They are filled with celebrities and testimonials affirming the perfection of the product or service. They have a strong impact on consumers, particularly those susceptible to impulse purchasing.

**Internist:** A medical doctor who specializes in the internal organs of the body, especially the stomach, intestines, and colon.

**Jejunum:** Middle section of small intestine, where most digestion occurs.

**Lumbar:** It is also called the lower back. There are five vertebrae that comprise this section of the spinal column.

**Manicurist:** A licensed professional who performs services in the beauty industry on the feet and hands, most commonly referred to as pedicures and manicures. Also performs reflexology.

**Masseur:** A man who is licensed to perform massage on all parts of the body. He usually does several different styles of massage; reflexology is only one of many.

**Masseuse:** A woman who is licensed to perform massage on all parts of the body. She usually does several different styles of massage; reflexology is only one of many.

**Meridian points:** These are the reflective centers found all over the body. These are centers of nerve fibers that send messages to and back from the brain. They control all the various parts of the body, internally and externally. There are 10 zones throughout the body, with 5 on the left side and 5 on the right. They are distributed from the top of the body to the bottom, from the front to the back. They encompass a 360° circle from any direction. They are also referred to as the reflex centers or points.

**Nondominant:** The side that the person does not use the most. A right-handed person's nondominant side is the left. In reflexology the nondominant side is accessed first because it responds better during the session.

**Nonlegitimate massage therapist:** It was common for prostitutes to use the title of massage therapist to gain customers. It was difficult for a legitimate therapist to gain respect in the community because of the widely used title. Among the licensed, legal professional masseuses, the term nonlegitimate became popular.

**OTC:** Common abbreviation for products sold over the counter, most often refers to drugs sold without a medical prescription. Examples: aspirin, antihistamines, and cough syrup.

**Ovary:** The female reproductive glands in which the ova and hormones that regulate female secondary sex characteristics develop.

**Ovulation:** The act of shedding the female eggs from the ovary.

**Peptic ulcer:** A specific kind of ulcer found in the walls of the stomach. The highly powerful acids of the stomach work to makc a hole in the lining of the stomach.

**Personal space:** The area around our bodies that extends from our head to the fingertips, when our arms are fully extended outward. We usually require permission to get close to another person when it is within these boundaries. It is usually offered unconditionally only to family members and special loved ones.

**Pharynx:** The part of the alimentary canal between the cavity of the mouth and the esophagus.

**Pineal gland:** It has an unknown function present in the brain of all vertebrates having a cranium, believed to be a vestigial sense organ.

**Pituitary gland:** A small, oval endocrine gland attached to the base of the brain and situated in a depression of the sphenoid bone; secretes several hormones.

**Prostate:** The muscular glandular organ that surrounds the urethra of males at the base of the bladder.

**Reflex center/points:** Also known as meridians.

**Reflexology:** The word itself has two parts. The root "reflex" and "ology." The second is easier to explain, because "ology" at the end of any word means "the study of." In the case of reflexology, it is the study of the reflexes. The use of the root "reflex" in the word reflexology refers to the "reaction" of the meridian points found throughout the body. These highly sensitive nerve endings send messages back to the brain. Through developed sensory pathways, they can tell what is going on inside the body. Another way to describe their ability to detect what is going on inside is to say that they act as a "reflex" to the internal system of the body. Therefore "reflexology" is the study of the reaction of the meridian points of the body. It is also the science of understanding what the meridians are all about. It is the exact method used to bring about balance to the internal system of the body by interceding and sending a new message back to the brain through the meridian points.

**Relay points:** Also known as meridian points.

**Shiatsu:** An ancient Chinese/Japanese method of massage. It means "finger pressure." The meridian points are accessed during this massage. Part of the acupressure massage system, it is the gentlest of all the massages.

**Sigmoid colon:** The last part of the colon system. It holds the fecal material for final release through the anus.

**Sodium pentothal:** A drug used to remove the sensation of pain by putting the patient to sleep. In actuality the drug is a poison that forces the brain to shut down and the patient loses consciousness. It must be administered intravenously (through a needle into the vein), and the patient's vital signs, heart rate, and blood pressure must be closely monitored.

**Solar plexus:** The area between the breast plate and above the diaphragm. It has a strong link to the pathway to the brain. Although not very well understood, it seems to have a significant response mechanism to a person feeling emotionally well balanced.

**Stethoscope:** A medical instrument used to hear the heartbeat and sound of air as it passes through the lungs.

**Stratum corneum:** The top of five layers that comprise the cells that make up the epidermal layer of the skin. It is the dead layer of tissue made up of keratin fibers that lies on the outer edge of the skin. It is the skin tissue that we see and feel when we touch our bodies. It is the driest part of the skin, containing little or no water.

**Sympathy pains:** When one person experiences similar discomfort or pain with another person. It often occurs for young first-time fathers-to-be while their partners are going through pregnancy.

**Testicle:** A male productive gland, either of two oval glands located in the scrotum.

**Thoracic:** This is the middle part of spinal column. There are twelve vertebrae in this region.

**Thymus:** A gland, resembling the appearance of a walnut, which is largely comprised of lymphoid tissue. In an embryo, it is used as the immune system. It lies in the thorax near the base of the neck and it produces T cells when lymphocytes pass through it.

**Thyroid:** Part of the endocrine system, located in the throat area. It produces a hormone called thyroxine which is primarily made up of iodine. It controls the body's weight through hormonal balance and metabolism and also regulates the oxygen level and heat production of the system on demand. It is the most important and largest gland of the entire endocrine system.

**Trades:** This is a way of doing business that does not cause you to spend cash. You work out an arrangement that allows you to receive a service or product in exchange for one of your services or products. It is so popular that organizations are set up all over the country that handle the process, called Barter USA.

**Transverse colon:** The middle portion of the colon that extends across the abdominal cavity. One of four parts of the colon.

**Ulcer:** A break in skin or mucous membrane with a loss of surface tissue. Sometimes festers with pus (a sign of infection). The entire digestive tract is susceptible to ulcers, including the stomach, the intestines, and the colon (all four sections).

**Uterus:** The portion of the oviduct in which the fertilized egg implants itself and develops or rests during prenatal development. Also called the womb in certain mammals.

# *Appendix B*

## REFLEXOLOGY
## SOURCES

These companies and schools provide hands-on training in reflexology.

### Digits International Reflexology Institute
27636 Ynez Road L-7 Siute #232,
Temecula, CA 92591
800-229-0225

This company has one of the most extensive educational programs of seminars and classes available on reflexology.

### The Academy of Healing Arts Massage and Facial Skin Care Inc.
3141 S. Military Trail, Lakeworth, FL 33463
407-967-0899

This company has classes on many different kinds of massage; reflexology is one of them.

### The Boston Institute of Esthetics
47 Spring Street, West Roxbury, MA 02132
617-323-0844

This company specializes in skin care classes, but reflexology is included in their training.

### The Conservatory of Esthetics
Midwest: 324 W. Touhy Avenue,
   Park Ridge, IL 60068
800-433-6650

West Coast: 8214 1/2 Melrose Avenue.,
   Los Angeles, CA 90046
800-433-6650

This school offers a wide variety of classes; reflexology is included at both locations.

### Von Lee International School of Esthetics Inc.
309 Reisterstown Road, Baltimore, MD 21208
800-437-5140

This licensing school offers reflexology as part of its advanced continuing education curriculum.

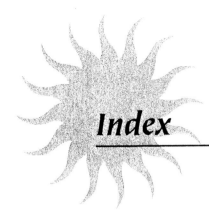

# *Index*

Intestines, 87, 91, 92, 120, 121
  *See also* Colon; Constipation;
    Flatulence; Small intestine
Iron supplements, 155
Irregularity, 118, 156
  *See also* Constipation

**J**
Japanese Shiatsu, 161
Jejunum, 120, 159
Joint offerings, 88, 150–151
Jones, Sally, 74–75

**K**
Karen (client), 96–98
Keratin, 162

**L**
Laguna Beach, 33–34
Laxatives, 120, 125
Left-handedness, 53
Licensing boards, 17, 28, 37–39, 53,
  59
Liver, 57
Lotions, 21
"Love Child" movement, 31
Lumbar vertebrae, 159
Lupus, 41

**M**
Male clients, 142–143
Male organs. *See* Prostate; Testicles
Manic/depressive tendencies, 112
Manicurists, 17, 25
  defined, 159
  foot manipulation by, 59
  hand manipulation by, 53
  licensing of, 38, 53
  nails of, 34, 35
  stylists and, 20–21, 22, 27–28
Marketing, 139–152
Masseuses/masseurs, 17, 18–20
  back treatment by, 76
  defined, 159
  foot manipulation by, 59
  freedom of, 28
  hand manipulation by, 53
  licensing of, 38

nails of, 34
personal contact with, 32–33
reflexology and, 4, 25, 117–118
Masturbation, 89
Medical doctors. *See* Physicians
Medical examinations, 4–5
Medical problems. *See* Diseases
Medical review boards, 42
Medical treatments
  for back problems, 75
  on Client History form, 12
  for constipation, 118
  for depression, 111
  for major organs, 55
  side effects of, 9–10
  for ulcers, 82
  *See also* Holistic health care
Medications
  for manic/depressive
    tendencies, 112
  pregnancy and, 84, 91
  records on, 133
  side effects of, 102, 118
  *See also* Over-the-counter
    medications
Menopause, 89, 90
Menstrual cramps, 89, 98–101
Menstruation. *See* Ovulation;
  Premenstrual syndrome
Mental health. *See* Depression;
  Mood swings
Meridian points
  defined, 4, 159
  of internal organs, 39, 42
  massage therapists and, 18
  pain at, 7–9, 130–131
  study of, 161
  sympathetic response of, 10
Metabolism, 82, 163
Mood swings, 91, 93, 94
Morning sickness, 84, 91, 92
Muscle reflexes, 4

**N**
Nail salons, 20, 21–22
Nails, 33–35
Nausea, 84, 101
Neck, 57, 103–104